COLOSTOMY DIET COOKBOOK

Nourishing Recipes and Essential Guidance for Optimal Health and Comfortable Living After Your Surgery

Craig Kante

Copyright © 2024 All rights reserved.

No part of this book may be reproduced or transmitted in any form or by any means, electronic or mechanical, including photocopying, recording, or by any information storage and retrieval system, without written permission from the author. The scanning, uploading, and distribution of this book via the internet or via any other means without the permission of the author is illegal and punishable by law. The author has made every effort to ensure the accuracy of the information contained in this book. However, the author cannot be held responsible for any errors or omissions.

Table of Contents

Introduction..7

Chapter 1
- Understanding Colostomy..9
- Dietary Guidelines for Colostomy Patients..................................11
- Foods to Avoid and Why..13
- Essential Nutrients for Colostomy Patients................................15

Breakfast Recipes
Banana Oatmeal...17
Apple Sauce Pancakes..18
Smoothie Bowl...19
Soft-Boiled Eggs..20
Cottage Cheese and Peaches...21
Quinoa Porridge...22
Blueberry Muffins..23
Pumpkin Bread..24
Avocado Toast..25
Rice Cakes with Cottage Cheese..26
Soft Fruit Salad..27
Porridge...28
Peach Yogurt Parfait...29
Egg Muffins..30
Soft Cheese Omelette..31
Peach Smoothie..32
Cinnamon Toast..33
Baked Oatmeal..34
Soft Cheese and Crackers...35
Egg and Cheese Quesadilla..36
Creamy Semolina..37

Poultry Recipes
Baked Chicken Breast..38
Chicken and Rice Soup..39
Chicken and Quinoa Salad..40
Poached Chicken..41
Lemon Herb Chicken...42

Chicken and Carrot Stew...........43
Chicken and Sweet Potato Bake...........44
Chicken and Broccoli Casserole...........45
Chicken Meatballs...........46
Chicken and Zucchini Skewers...........47
Chicken and Spinach Frittata...........48
Chicken and Pumpkin Stew...........49
Chicken and Cauliflower Mash...........50
Chicken and Apple Salad...........51
Chicken and Green Bean Stir-Fry...........52
Chicken and Butternut Squash Bake...........53
Chicken and Tomato Pasta...........54
Chicken and Pea Risotto...........55
Chicken and Carrot Puree...........56
Chicken and Rice Paper Rolls...........57
Chicken and Spinach Soup...........58
Chicken and Mashed Potatoes...........59
Baked Turkey Breast...........60
Turkey and Vegetable Soup...........61
Turkey and Quinoa Salad...........62
Turkey and Sweet Potato Hash...........63
Turkey Meatballs...........64

Beef and Pork Recipes
Beef and Rice Soup...........65
Beef Stew...........66
Ground Beef and Quinoa Bowl...........67
Beef Meatballs...........68
Pork and Rice Soup...........69
Pork Stew...........70
Pork Meatballs...........71
Pork and Apricot Salad...........72
Pork and Vegetable Bake...........73
Pork and Mushroom Casserole...........74
Pork and Carrot Salad...........75
Pork and Vegetable Soup...........76
Pork and Spinach Soup...........77
Pork and Soft Vegetable Casserole...........78
Beef and Apricot Salad...........79
Beef and Vegetable Bake...........80
Beef and Pumpkin Mash...........81
Beef and Mashed Potatoes...........82
Beef and Carrot Puree...........83

Fish and Seafood Recipes

Baked Salmon..84
Grilled Cod..85
Baked Tilapia..86
Salmon Cakes...87
Fish Tacos...88
Cod and Sweet Potato Bake..89
Salmon and Spinach Frittata..90
Grilled Halibut...91
Cod and Bell Pepper Stir-Fry...92
Salmon and Butternut Squash Stew..93
Grilled Sole..94
Grilled Mahi Mahi...95
Baked Flounder...96
Shrimp and Rice Soup...97
Grilled Shrimp Skewers...98
Baked Scallops..99
Shrimp and Rice Casserole..100
Grilled Scallops with Rice...101
Grilled Shrimp with Bell Peppers..102
Shrimp and Zucchini Soup...103

Snacks & Sides Recipes

Yogurt with Honey...104
Rice Cakes with Avocado...105
Oatmeal Cookies..106
Banana Bread..107
Boiled Carrot Sticks...108
Peanut Butter and Banana Sandwich....................................109
Smoothie Popsicles..110
Fruit Smoothie Bowl..111
Mashed Potatoes..112
Steamed Carrots...113
Boiled Zucchini...114
Steamed Spinach...115
Soft Polenta...116
Creamed Corn...117
Rice Noodles...118

10-WEEK MEAL PLAN..119

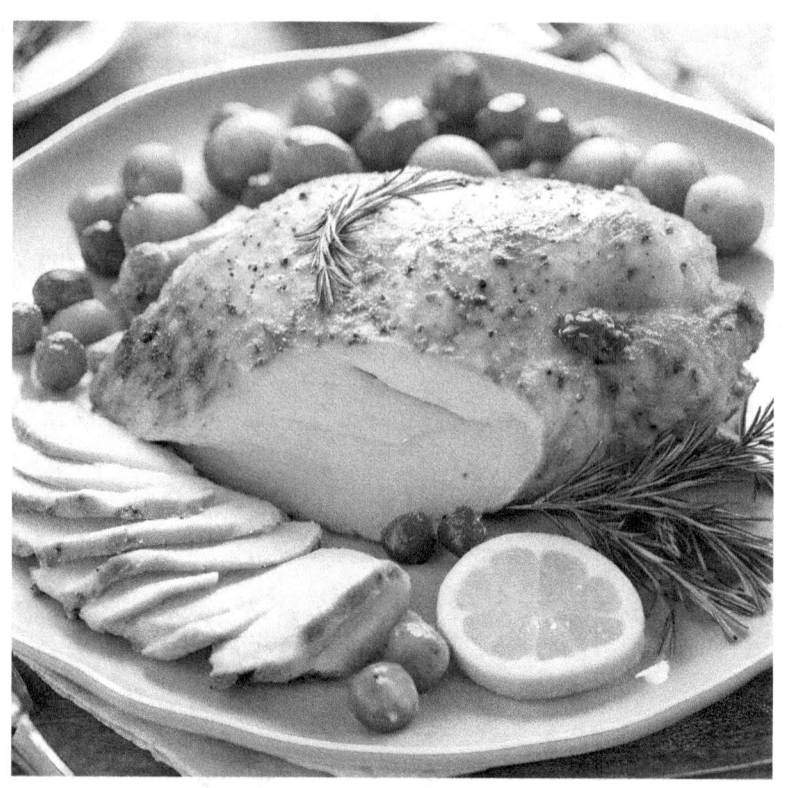

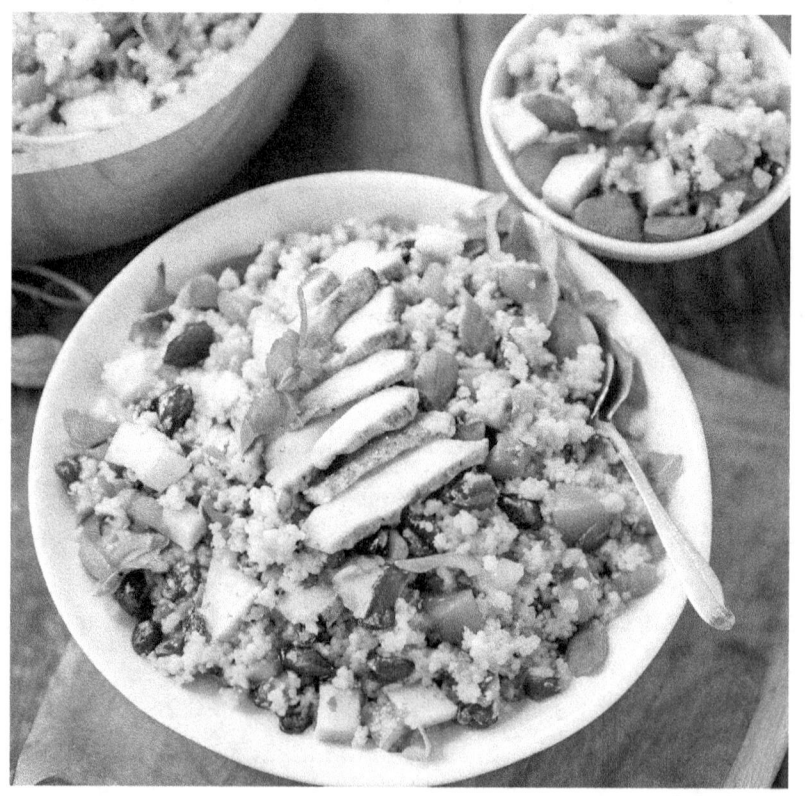

To show our appreciation for your purchase, we're delighted to offer you these special bonuses as a heartfelt thank you.

1. A Food Tracker Journal
2. Downloadable E-BOOK featuring full-color images of finished recipes

Introduction

Navigating life after a colostomy can be a profound challenge, especially when it comes to adapting your diet. Understanding what to eat, how to prepare it, and when to consume meals can become overwhelming. That's where the "Colostomy Diet Cookbook" comes in—your compassionate guide to reclaiming culinary enjoyment and nutritional balance. After a colostomy, you might feel that your food choices are severely limited, but this cookbook is designed to dispel that myth, providing you with a wide array of tasty, nutritious, and easy-to-prepare recipes. Whether you are a novice in the kitchen or a seasoned chef, this book ensures that a colostomy does not restrict your enjoyment of food but rather opens a new door to exploring healthy and delicious eating.

The recipes in this cookbook are more than just suitable for a colostomy; they are crafted to enhance your health and ensure that your digestive system functions optimally. We understand the delicate balance required to manage digestion and avoid complications such as blockages or dehydration. Therefore, each recipe is designed with the right blend of fiber, hydration, and nutrients to support your body's needs and promote well-being. "Eating well" takes on a whole new meaning in the context of living with a colostomy. It's not just about the nutrients and the numbers—it's about enhancing your quality of life, stabilizing your energy levels, and providing you with meal options that are both satisfying and safe. The **Colostomy Diet Cookbook** includes a variety of recipes—from hearty breakfasts to sumptuous dinners and delightful desserts—that cater to personal tastes and dietary requirements while considering the unique needs of individuals with a colostomy. This cookbook also serves as an educational resource, offering insights into how different foods can affect your colostomy. You'll find practical advice on how to manage common issues like gas, odor, and pouch management through dietary choices. Our goal is to empower you with the knowledge and culinary skills to manage your health proactively. Moreover, the "Colostomy Diet Cookbook" is infused with stories from people just like you—those who have adapted to life with a colostomy and thrived. These personal anecdotes add a layer of community and support, reminding you that you are not alone on this journey. They share their trials and triumphs, giving practical advice and emotional encouragement.

Living with a colostomy may have changed the way you live, but it doesn't have to define your life. This cookbook is a celebration of the adaptability and resilience of the human spirit, a testament to the fact that a fulfilling life is possible post-surgery. With this book in your kitchen, you are equipped not just to cope, but to thrive. It's not just about surviving; it's about flourishing—with every meal and every recipe providing you the opportunity to live your life to the fullest.

Set out on this culinary journey with the **Colostomy Diet Cookbook** as your companion. Embrace the art of cooking with confidence and joy, and let food be your ally in the path to recovery and beyond. Here's to new beginnings and a healthier, happier you!

Chapter 1

Understanding Colostomy

A colostomy is a life-changing procedure that, for many, can bring a mix of relief, fear, and uncertainty. It is a surgical operation where an opening, known as a stoma, is created in the abdomen to divert the colon's end to an external bag. This procedure is often necessary for individuals suffering from severe bowel diseases, cancer, or traumatic injury. Understanding colostomy is essential for patients and their loved ones, as it can transform how one lives, eats, and views daily activities. The journey towards accepting and adapting to a colostomy can be emotionally challenging. Initially, the thought of living with a stoma can be daunting, and it's not uncommon to feel overwhelmed. You may ask yourself, *"Why me?"* or worry about how your life will change. It's important to remember that these feelings are completely natural. Embracing this new reality often requires time, patience, and support from family, friends, and healthcare professionals. Living with a colostomy means making adjustments, particularly in diet and lifestyle. It's not just about managing a new way to eliminate waste; it's about ensuring your body gets the right nutrients while avoiding foods that might cause discomfort or complications. For many, the journey begins with trial and error, discovering which foods sit well and which don't. This can be frustrating, but with guidance and perseverance, you will find a balance that works for you.

Diet plays a crucial role in managing life with a colostomy. Certain foods might cause blockages, excess gas, or unpleasant odors, making social situations or even mealtime a source of anxiety. However, learning to navigate these challenges can lead to a more confident and fulfilling life. Your diet will likely include plenty of water, easy-to-digest foods, and a careful selection of fiber. Remember, you are not alone in this; many resources and communities are available to help you adjust.

One of the most empowering steps in understanding colostomy is recognizing the incredible resilience and adaptability of the human spirit. Many people with colostomies lead active, fulfilling lives, engaging in sports, traveling, and pursuing their passions. The key is to focus on what you can do rather than what you can't. Support groups can be invaluable, providing a space to share experiences, tips, and encouragement. These communities remind you that there's a whole network of individuals who understand your journey.

Dietary Guidelines for Colostomy Patients

Navigating life after a colostomy can be a complex journey, especially when it comes to diet. The foods you eat play a crucial role in your overall well-being and can significantly impact how well you manage your colostomy. While adjusting to new dietary guidelines may seem overwhelming at first, it's also an opportunity to explore nourishing meals that keep you feeling your best and living life to the fullest. One of the most important aspects of a colostomy-friendly diet is understanding the balance between fiber intake and digestibility. **Fiber** is essential for healthy digestion, but after a colostomy, too much fiber can cause blockages, while too little can lead to constipation. It's all about finding that sweet spot. Start with low-fiber foods like white rice, pasta, and peeled fruits and vegetables, and gradually reintroduce higher-fiber options as you learn what your body can handle.

Hydration is another critical component. Colostomy patients are more prone to dehydration because their bodies may absorb less water from their food. Drinking plenty of fluids, especially water, is vital. Aim for at least eight glasses a day, and consider incorporating hydrating foods like cucumbers, melons, and soups into your diet. Remember, staying hydrated helps maintain healthy digestion and overall bodily function.
Gas and odor control are common concerns for colostomy patients. Certain foods can exacerbate these issues, so it's wise to be mindful of your choices. Foods like beans, onions, carbonated beverages, and cruciferous vegetables (such as broccoli and cabbage) may increase gas production. While these foods are nutritious, they might need to be limited or introduced slowly. Additionally, consuming yogurt or other probiotic-rich foods can help balance your gut bacteria, potentially reducing gas and odor.

Eating small, frequent meals can also be beneficial. Large meals can be harder to digest and may cause discomfort. Instead, try having five to six smaller meals throughout the day. This approach can make it easier for your digestive system to process food and can help you maintain consistent energy levels.

It's also crucial to chew your food thoroughly. This simple step aids digestion and can prevent blockages. Take your time while eating, savoring each bite, and enjoying the flavors and textures of your meal. This mindful eating practice not only helps with digestion but also enhances your overall dining experience. Support from dietitians and nutritionists can be invaluable. These professionals can provide personalized advice based on your specific needs and preferences. They can help you create a balanced diet plan that supports your health and lifestyle, making the transition smoother and more manageable.

Living with a colostomy doesn't mean you have to give up the joy of eating delicious food. It's about learning to listen to your body and making informed choices that support your health. As you adapt to these dietary guidelines, you'll likely find a new appreciation for food and how it fuels your body. Remember, every step you take towards understanding and managing your diet is a step towards reclaiming your confidence and living your life to the fullest. Embrace this journey with patience and kindness towards yourself. With time, the dietary changes will become second nature, and you'll discover that living with a colostomy can be a fulfilling and empowered experience.

Foods to Avoid and Why

High-Fiber Foods
While fiber is essential for digestive health, too much can lead to blockages for colostomy patients. Foods high in insoluble fiber, such as raw vegetables, corn, popcorn, nuts, seeds, and the skins of fruits and vegetables, can be particularly problematic. These foods pass through the digestive system relatively unchanged, which can cause obstructions in the stoma. To avoid these complications, it's best to introduce fiber gradually into your diet and opt for soluble fiber sources like oats, bananas, and applesauce, which are easier to digest.

Gas-Producing Foods
Living with a colostomy often involves managing gas production, as excess gas can be uncomfortable and embarrassing. Certain foods are notorious for causing gas, including beans, lentils, broccoli, cabbage, onions, and carbonated beverages. These foods contain complex carbohydrates and fibers that are fermented by bacteria in the colon, producing gas as a byproduct. While these foods are nutritious, it's wise to consume them in moderation and observe how your body reacts. Keeping a food diary can help identify specific triggers, allowing you to adjust your diet accordingly.

Odor-Causing Foods
Odor management is another critical aspect of living with a colostomy. Foods such as garlic, onions, fish, eggs, and certain spices can produce strong odors that may be bothersome. Although these foods are flavorful and healthy, their impact on odor can be significant. To mitigate this, you can incorporate odor-reducing foods like parsley, yogurt, and cranberry juice into your diet. These foods can help neutralize odors and make social situations more comfortable.

Difficult-to-Digest Foods
Some foods are simply hard to digest and can cause discomfort or blockages. Tough meats, dried fruits, coconut, and high-fat or fried foods fall into this category. These foods take longer to break down and can strain your digestive system. Instead, opt for tender, lean meats, and well-cooked fruits and vegetables. These alternatives are easier on your system and still provide the necessary nutrients for your health.

Sugar Alcohols
Sugar alcohols, found in many sugar-free products like gum, candy, and some processed foods, can cause bloating, gas, and diarrhea. These compounds are not fully absorbed by the body, leading to fermentation by bacteria in the intestines. Reading labels and avoiding foods containing ingredients like sorbitol, mannitol, and xylitol can help prevent these uncomfortable side effects.

Spicy Foods
While many enjoy the heat and flavor of spicy foods, they can irritate the digestive tract and cause increased output from the stoma. If you're sensitive to spicy foods, it's best to avoid them or consume them in moderation. Opt for milder seasonings and herbs to flavor your meals without causing irritation.

Practical Tips
Navigating dietary restrictions can feel daunting, but with time and patience, you'll learn what works best for your body. Keeping a food diary to track what you eat and how it affects you can be incredibly helpful. Consulting with a dietitian can also provide personalized guidance and support. Remember, you're not alone in this journey. Many others have successfully adapted to life with a colostomy, and with the right information and mindset, you can too.

Essential Nutrients for Colostomy Patients

Protein: The Building Block of Healing
Protein is crucial for tissue repair and wound healing, making it an essential nutrient for colostomy patients. Surgery and recovery increase the body's demand for protein, which helps repair tissues, build muscles, and support the immune system. Lean meats like chicken, turkey, and fish are excellent sources, as are plant-based options such as tofu, lentils, and beans. Including a variety of protein-rich foods in your diet can help ensure you're getting enough to support your recovery and health.

Hydration: The Lifeline of Digestive Health
Staying hydrated is paramount for colostomy patients. Adequate fluid intake helps prevent dehydration, which can be more common due to changes in the digestive system. Water, herbal teas, and clear broths are excellent choices. Hydrating foods like cucumbers, oranges, and watermelon can also contribute to your fluid intake. Sipping fluids throughout the day rather than consuming large amounts at once can help your body maintain optimal hydration levels.

Electrolytes: The Balancers of Body Function
Electrolytes such as sodium, potassium, and magnesium are vital for maintaining fluid balance and proper muscle function. Colostomy patients may experience fluctuations in electrolyte levels, particularly if they have increased output from the stoma. Bananas, oranges, and leafy greens are rich in potassium, while nuts, seeds, and whole grains provide magnesium. Including a variety of these foods in your diet can help maintain balanced electrolyte levels.

Fiber: The Gentle Guide to Digestion
Fiber is essential for promoting healthy digestion, but finding the right balance is crucial for colostomy patients. While too much fiber can cause blockages, too little can lead to constipation. Soluble fiber, found in oats, bananas, and apples, is gentler on the digestive system and helps regulate bowel movements. Gradually incorporating fiber into your diet and observing how your body reacts can help you find a comfortable balance.

Vitamins and Minerals: The Foundation of Vitality
A well-rounded diet rich in vitamins and minerals supports overall health and vitality. Vitamin C, found in citrus fruits and strawberries, aids in wound healing and boosts the immune system. Vitamin A, present in carrots and sweet potatoes, supports skin health and vision. B vitamins, abundant in whole grains and leafy greens, play a crucial role in energy production and nerve function. Ensuring a colorful variety of fruits and vegetables on your plate can help you meet your nutritional needs.

Iron: The Energizer of the Body
Iron is essential for producing hemoglobin, which carries oxygen throughout the body. After a colostomy, it's important to prevent iron deficiency, which can lead to fatigue and weakness. Lean red meat, poultry, fish, and plant-based sources like lentils and spinach are excellent sources of iron. Pairing iron-rich foods with vitamin C-rich foods can enhance absorption, ensuring you get the most benefit from your diet.

Calcium and Vitamin D: The Guardians of Bone Health
Calcium and vitamin D are crucial for maintaining strong bones and teeth. Dairy products, fortified plant-based milks, and leafy greens provide calcium, while sunlight exposure and foods like fatty fish and fortified cereals offer vitamin D. These nutrients work together to support bone health, which is especially important if your activity levels have changed post-surgery.

Personalization and Support
Every individual's nutritional needs are unique, especially when adjusting to life with a colostomy. Working with a dietitian can help tailor your diet to meet your specific needs and preferences. They can provide personalized guidance, ensuring you get the essential nutrients your body requires.

Adjusting to a new diet after a colostomy can be a journey filled with trial and error, but it's also a path to discovering how to nurture your body with compassion and care. Embrace each step with patience and kindness towards yourself. Celebrate the small victories, like finding a meal that makes you feel good or discovering a new favorite food. Remember, you're not alone on this journey—there's a whole community of support to help you along the way.

Breakfast Recipes

1. Banana Oatmeal
Ingredients
- 1 cup rolled oats
- 2 cups water or milk (dairy or plant-based)
- 1 ripe banana, mashed
- 1 tablespoon honey or maple syrup
- 1/2 teaspoon ground cinnamon
- A pinch of salt
- Optional toppings: sliced banana, nuts, seeds, or berries

Instructions
1. In a medium saucepan, bring the water or milk to a boil.
2. Add the oats and a pinch of salt, then reduce the heat to medium and simmer for 5 minutes, stirring occasionally.
3. Stir in the mashed banana, honey or maple syrup, and ground cinnamon. Continue to cook for another 2-3 minutes until the oats are soft and creamy.
4. Remove from heat and let it sit for a minute to thicken.
5. Serve hot, topped with optional sliced banana, nuts, seeds, or berries.

Nutrition Info per Serving
- Calories: 220
- Protein: 5g
- Fat: 3g
- Carbohydrates: 45g
- Fiber: 5g
- Sugars: 12g

Serves
2

Cooking Time
10 minutes

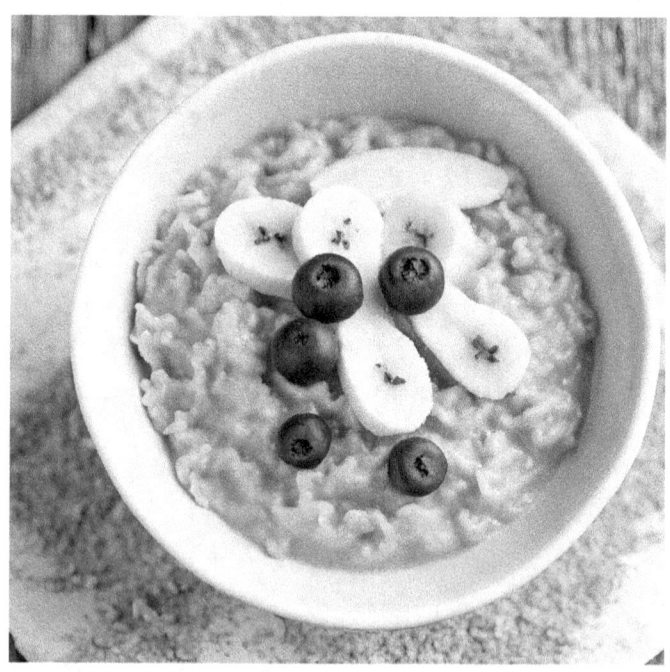

2. Apple Sauce Pancakes

Ingredients
- 1 cup whole wheat flour
- 1 tablespoon baking powder
- 1/2 teaspoon ground cinnamon
- 1/4 teaspoon salt
- 1 cup unsweetened applesauce
- 1/2 cup milk (dairy or plant-based)
- 1 large egg
- 1 tablespoon honey or maple syrup
- 1 teaspoon vanilla extract
- Cooking spray or oil for the pan

Instructions
1. In a large bowl, whisk together the flour, baking powder, ground cinnamon, and salt.
2. In another bowl, mix the applesauce, milk, egg, honey or maple syrup, and vanilla extract until well combined.
3. Pour the wet ingredients into the dry ingredients and stir until just combined. Do not overmix.
4. Heat a non-stick skillet or griddle over medium heat and lightly grease with cooking spray or oil.
5. Pour 1/4 cup of batter for each pancake onto the skillet. Cook until bubbles form on the surface, then flip and cook until golden brown on the other side, about 2-3 minutes per side.
6. Serve warm, optionally topped with extra applesauce or a drizzle of honey.

Nutrition Info per Serving
- Calories: 150
- Protein: 4g
- Fat: 2g
- Carbohydrates: 30g
- Fiber: 3g
- Sugars: 10g

Serves
4

Cooking Time
20 minutes

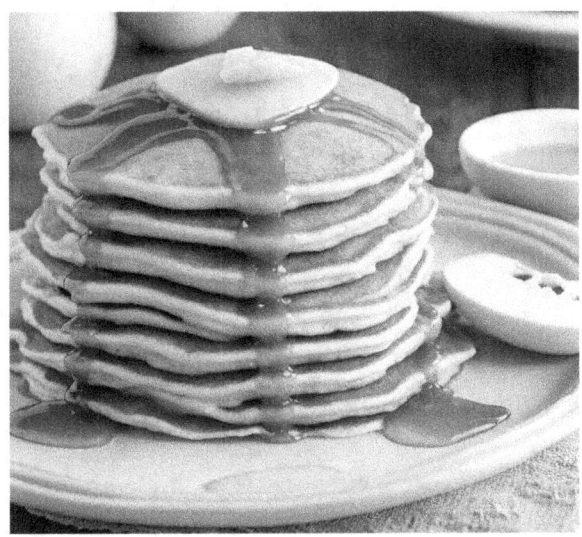

3. Smoothie Bowl

Ingredients
- 1 cup frozen berries (strawberries, blueberries, raspberries)
- 1 frozen banana
- 1/2 cup plain Greek yogurt or plant-based yogurt
- 1/4 cup milk (dairy or plant-based)
- 1 tablespoon honey or maple syrup (optional)
- Toppings: fresh fruit, granola, chia seeds, nuts

Instructions
1. In a blender, combine the frozen berries, frozen banana, yogurt, and milk. Blend until smooth and thick. Add honey or maple syrup if desired for sweetness.
2. Pour the smoothie into a bowl.
3. Top with fresh fruit, granola, chia seeds, or nuts as desired.
4. Serve immediately.

Nutrition Info per Serving
- Calories: 250
- Protein: 8g
- Fat: 4g
- Carbohydrates: 50g
- Fiber: 8g
- Sugars: 30g

Serves
2

Cooking Time
5 minutes

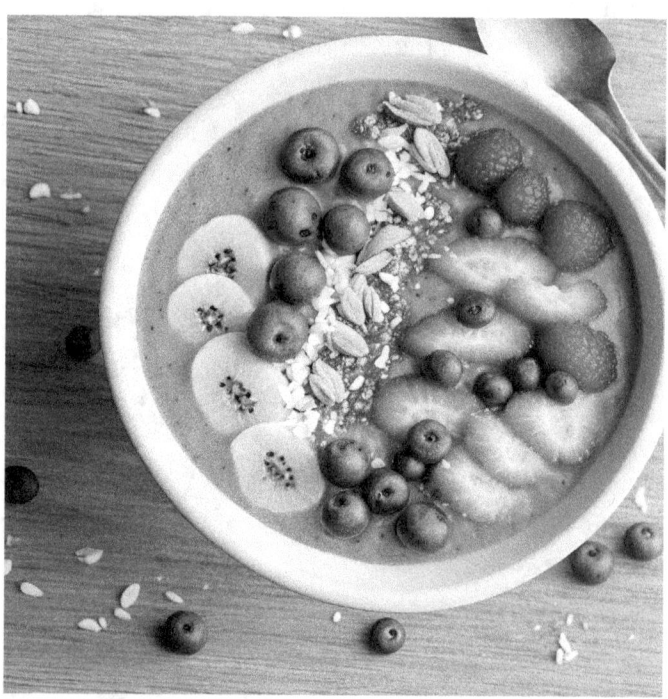

4. Soft-Boiled Eggs

Ingredients
- 4 large eggs
- Salt and pepper to taste

Instructions
1. Bring a medium saucepan of water to a rolling boil.
2. Carefully lower the eggs into the boiling water using a spoon.
3. Reduce the heat to maintain a gentle boil and cook the eggs for 6-7 minutes for a soft center.
4. While the eggs are cooking, prepare a bowl of ice water.
5. Once the eggs are done, transfer them immediately to the ice water to stop the cooking process. Let them sit for a couple of minutes.
6. Gently tap the eggs on a hard surface to crack the shell, then peel.
7. Serve the soft-boiled eggs with a sprinkle of salt and pepper.

Nutrition Info per Serving
- Calories: 70
- Protein: 6g
- Fat: 5g
- Carbohydrates: 1g
- Fiber: 0g
- Sugars: 0g

Serves
4

Cooking Time
10 minutes

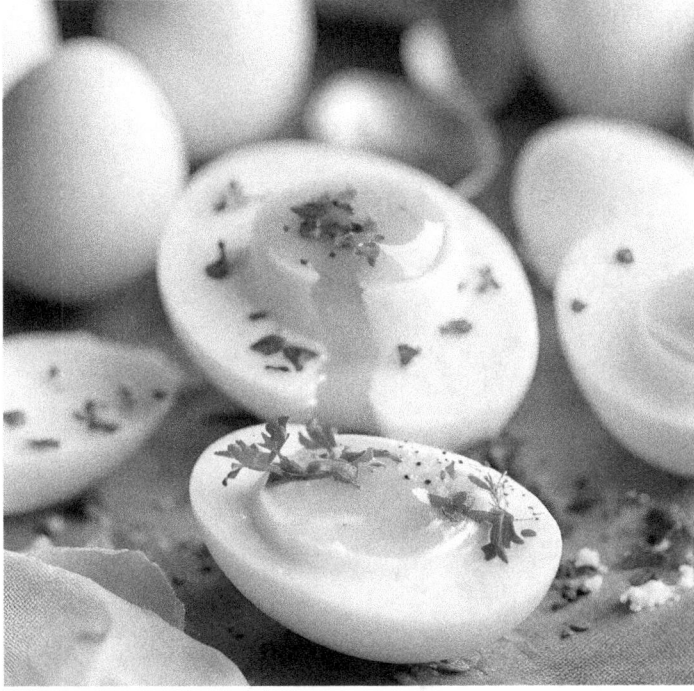

5. Cottage Cheese and Peaches

Ingredients
- 1 cup low-fat cottage cheese
- 1 large peach, sliced (or 1 cup canned peaches in juice, drained)
- 1 tablespoon honey or maple syrup (optional)
- 1/4 teaspoon ground cinnamon

Instructions
1. Place the cottage cheese in a bowl.
2. Arrange the peach slices on top of the cottage cheese.
3. Drizzle with honey or maple syrup, if desired.
4. Sprinkle with ground cinnamon.
5. Serve immediately.

Nutrition Info per Serving
- Calories: 150
- Protein: 14g
- Fat: 2g
- Carbohydrates: 20g
- Fiber: 2g
- Sugars: 12g

Serves
2

Cooking Time
5 minutes

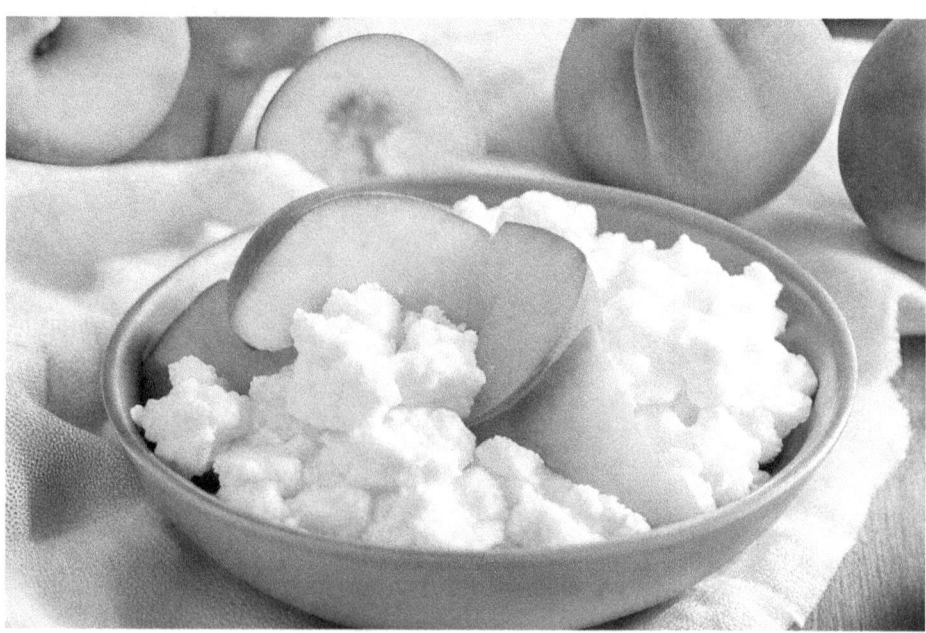

6. Quinoa Porridge

Ingredients
- 1 cup quinoa, rinsed
- 2 cups water
- 1 cup milk (dairy or plant-based)
- 1 tablespoon honey or maple syrup
- 1 teaspoon vanilla extract
- 1/2 teaspoon ground cinnamon
- Optional toppings: fresh fruit, nuts, seeds

Instructions
1. In a medium saucepan, bring the quinoa and water to a boil.
2. Reduce the heat to low, cover, and simmer for 15 minutes, or until the quinoa is tender and the water is absorbed.
3. Stir in the milk, honey or maple syrup, vanilla extract, and ground cinnamon.
4. Cook for another 5 minutes, stirring occasionally, until the porridge is creamy.
5. Remove from heat and let it sit for a minute to thicken.
6. Serve warm, topped with optional fresh fruit, nuts, or seeds.

Nutrition Info per Serving
- Calories: 230
- Protein: 7g
- Fat: 4g
- Carbohydrates: 40g
- Fiber: 3g
- Sugars: 10g

Serves
4

Cooking Time
25 minutes

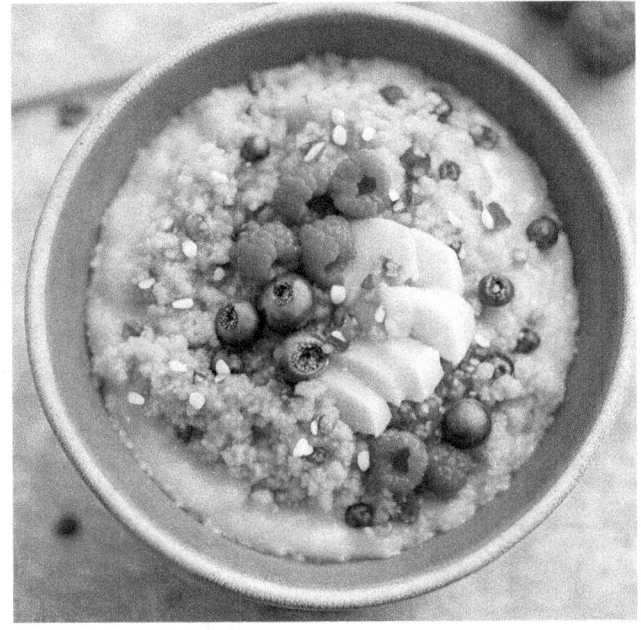

7. Blueberry Muffins

Ingredients
- 1 1/2 cups all-purpose flour
- 1/2 cup whole wheat flour
- 1 tablespoon baking powder
- 1/2 teaspoon salt
- 1/2 cup granulated sugar
- 1/2 cup unsweetened applesauce
- 1 large egg
- 1 cup milk (dairy or plant-based)
- 1 teaspoon vanilla extract
- 1 cup fresh or frozen blueberries

Instructions
1. Preheat the oven to 375°F (190°C). Line a muffin tin with paper liners.
2. In a large bowl, whisk together the flours, baking powder, salt, and sugar.
3. In another bowl, mix the applesauce, egg, milk, and vanilla extract until well combined.
4. Pour the wet ingredients into the dry ingredients and stir until just combined. Do not overmix.
5. Gently fold in the blueberries.
6. Divide the batter evenly among the muffin cups.
7. Bake for 20-25 minutes, or until a toothpick inserted into the center of a muffin comes out clean.
8. Allow the muffins to cool in the tin for 5 minutes, then transfer to a wire rack to cool completely.

Nutrition Info per Serving
- Calories: 130
- Protein: 3g
- Fat: 2g
- Carbohydrates: 26g
- Fiber: 2g
- Sugars: 10g

Serves
12 muffins

Cooking Time
30 minutes

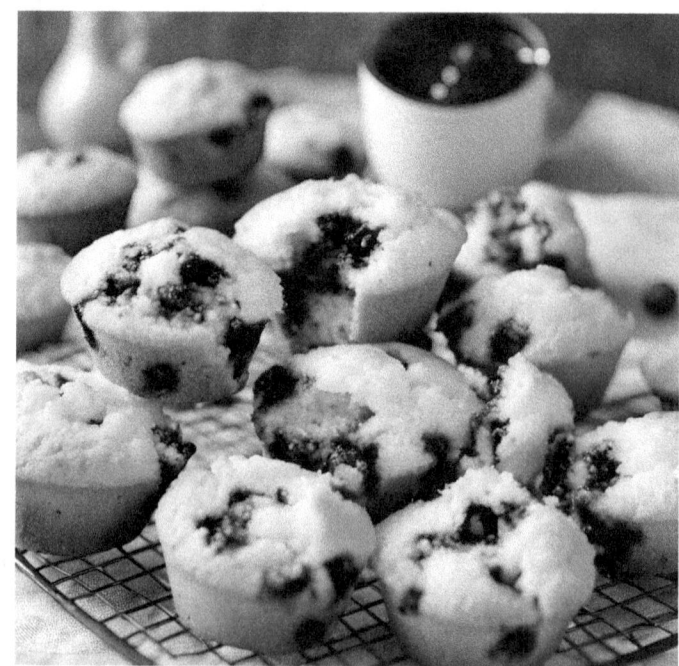

8. Pumpkin Bread
Ingredients
- 1 3/4 cups all-purpose flour
- 1/2 teaspoon baking powder
- 1/2 teaspoon baking soda
- 1/2 teaspoon salt
- 1 teaspoon ground cinnamon
- 1/2 teaspoon ground nutmeg
- 1/2 teaspoon ground ginger
- 1/4 teaspoon ground cloves
- 1 cup canned pumpkin puree
- 1/2 cup granulated sugar
- 1/2 cup brown sugar
- 1/2 cup vegetable oil
- 2 large eggs
- 1 teaspoon vanilla extract

Instructions
1. Preheat the oven to 350°F (175°C). Grease a 9x5-inch loaf pan.
2. In a large bowl, whisk together the flour, baking powder, baking soda, salt, cinnamon, nutmeg, ginger, and cloves.
3. In another bowl, mix the pumpkin puree, granulated sugar, brown sugar, oil, eggs, and vanilla extract until smooth.
4. Pour the wet ingredients into the dry ingredients and stir until just combined. Do not overmix.
5. Pour the batter into the prepared loaf pan.
6. Bake for 55-60 minutes, or until a toothpick inserted into the center comes out clean.
7. Allow the bread to cool in the pan for 10 minutes, then transfer to a wire rack to cool completely.

Nutrition Info per Serving
- Calories: 180
- Protein: 3g
- Fat: 8g
- Carbohydrates: 25g
- Fiber: 1g
- Sugars: 15g

Serves
10 slices

Cooking Time
70 minutes

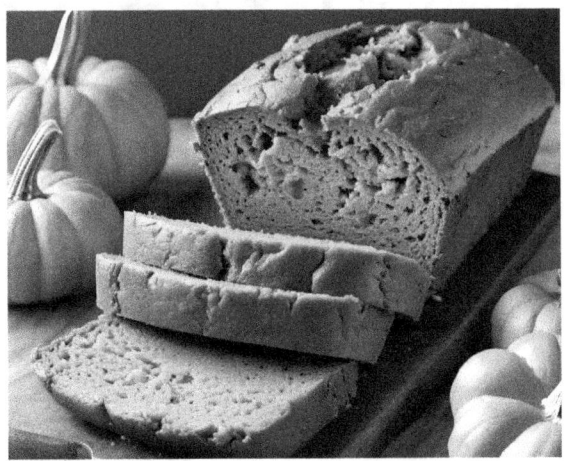

9. Avocado Toast

Ingredients
- 2 slices whole-grain bread
- 1 ripe avocado
- 1/2 lemon, juiced
- Salt and pepper to taste
- Optional toppings: cherry tomatoes, radishes, arugula, red pepper flakes

Instructions
1. Toast the bread slices to your desired level of crispiness.
2. In a bowl, mash the avocado with the lemon juice, salt, and pepper.
3. Spread the mashed avocado evenly onto the toasted bread.
4. Add optional toppings like cherry tomatoes, radishes, arugula, or red pepper flakes.
5. Serve immediately.

Nutrition Info per Serving
- Calories: 250
- Protein: 6g
- Fat: 15g
- Carbohydrates: 24g
- Fiber: 7g
- Sugars: 2g

Serves
2

Cooking Time
5 minutes

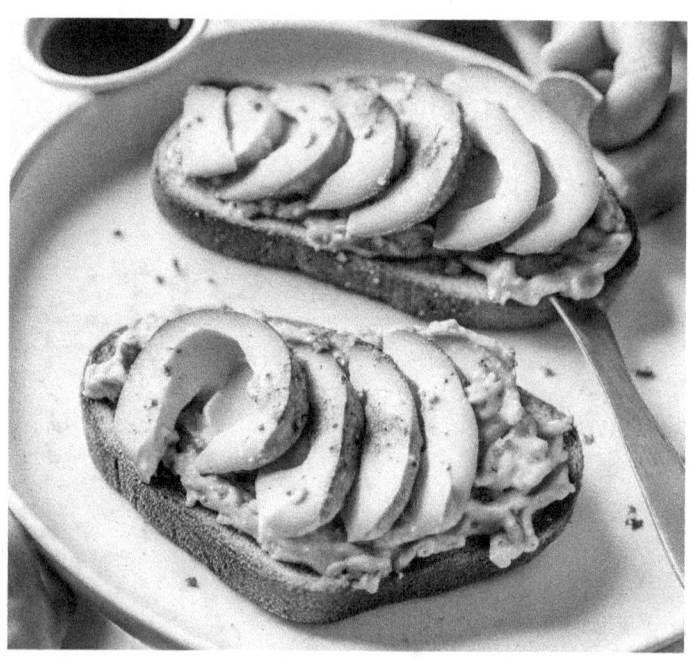

10. Rice Cakes with Cottage Cheese

Ingredients
- 4 plain rice cakes
- 1 cup low-fat cottage cheese
- 1/2 cup sliced cucumber
- 1/2 cup sliced cherry tomatoes
- Salt and pepper to taste
- Optional herbs: fresh dill, parsley, or chives

Instructions
1. Spread an even layer of cottage cheese on each rice cake.
2. Top with sliced cucumber and cherry tomatoes.
3. Sprinkle with salt and pepper to taste.
4. Garnish with optional fresh herbs if desired.
5. Serve immediately.

Nutrition Info per Serving
- Calories: 120
- Protein: 8g
- Fat: 2g
- Carbohydrates: 18g
- Fiber: 1g
- Sugars: 3g

Serves
4

Cooking Time
5 minutes

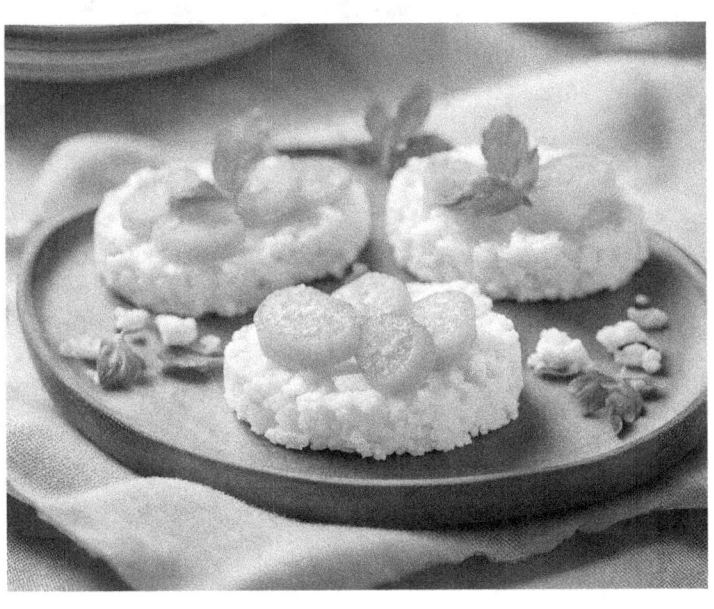

11. Soft Fruit Salad

Ingredients
- 1 cup ripe strawberries, hulled and sliced
- 1 cup ripe blueberries
- 1 ripe banana, sliced
- 1 cup ripe peach, diced (or canned peaches in juice, drained)
- 1 tablespoon honey or maple syrup
- 1 teaspoon lemon juice

Instructions
1. In a large bowl, combine the strawberries, blueberries, banana, and peach.
2. Drizzle with honey or maple syrup and lemon juice.
3. Gently toss to combine.
4. Serve immediately or chill in the refrigerator until ready to serve.

Nutrition Info per Serving
- Calories: 120
- Protein: 1g
- Fat: 0g
- Carbohydrates: 31g
- Fiber: 4g
- Sugars: 21g

Serves
4

Cooking Time
5 minutes

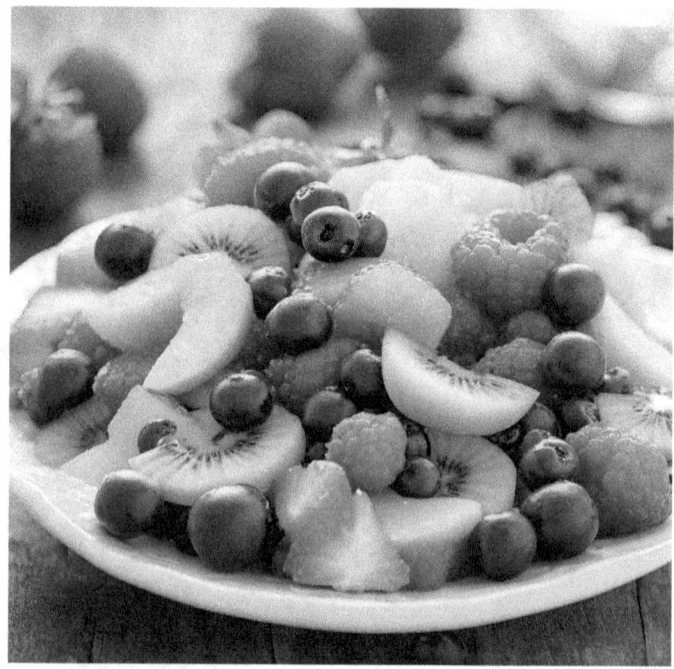

12. Porridge
Ingredients
- 1 cup rolled oats
- 2 cups water or milk (dairy or plant-based)
- 1 tablespoon honey or maple syrup
- 1/2 teaspoon ground cinnamon

Instructions
1. In a medium saucepan, bring the water or milk to a boil.
2. Add the oats and reduce the heat to medium. Simmer for 5 minutes, stirring occasionally.
3. Stir in the honey or maple syrup and ground cinnamon. Cook for another 2-3 minutes until the oats are soft and creamy.
4. Remove from heat and let it sit for a minute to thicken.
5. Serve hot.

Nutrition Info per Serving
- Calories: 220
- Protein: 5g
- Fat: 3g
- Carbohydrates: 45g
- Fiber: 4g
- Sugars: 12g

Serves
2

Cooking Time
10 minutes

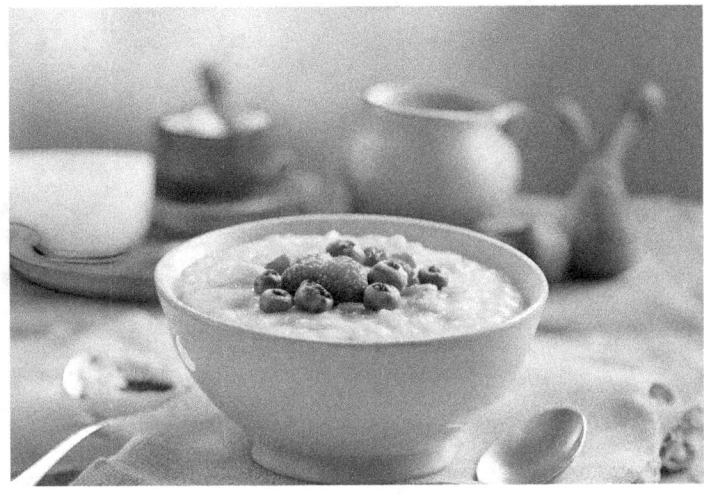

13. Peach Yogurt Parfait

Ingredients
- 2 cups plain Greek yogurt or plant-based yogurt
- 2 ripe peaches, diced (or canned peaches in juice, drained)
- 1/4 cup granola
- 1 tablespoon honey or maple syrup

Instructions
1. In two serving glasses or bowls, layer half of the yogurt.
2. Add a layer of diced peaches.
3. Add another layer of yogurt.
4. Top with remaining diced peaches and granola.
5. Drizzle with honey or maple syrup.
6. Serve immediately.

Nutrition Info per Serving
- Calories: 250
- Protein: 14g
- Fat: 5g
- Carbohydrates: 40g
- Fiber: 2g
- Sugars: 25g

Serves
2

Cooking Time
5 minutes

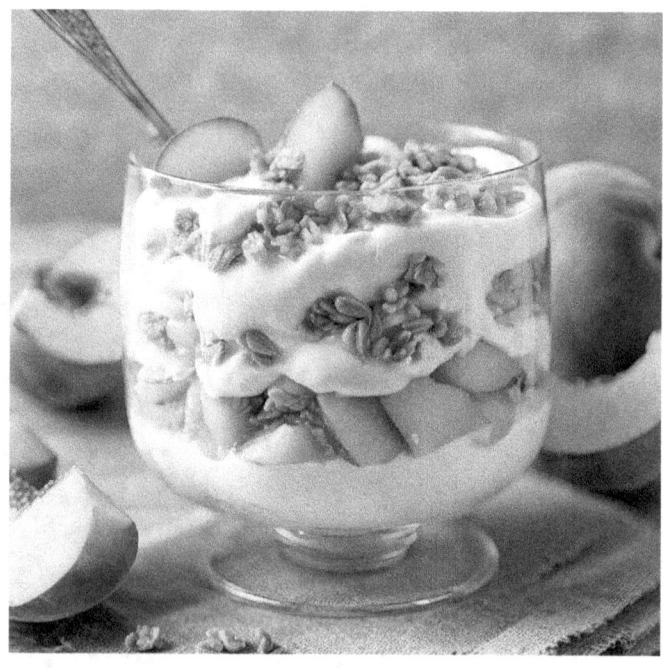

14. Egg Muffins

Ingredients
- 6 large eggs
- 1/4 cup milk (dairy or plant-based)
- 1/2 cup diced bell peppers
- 1/2 cup chopped spinach
- 1/4 cup shredded cheese
- 1/2 teaspoon ground paprika

Instructions
1. Preheat the oven to 350°F (175°C). Grease a muffin tin.
2. In a bowl, whisk together the eggs and milk.
3. Stir in the bell peppers, spinach, cheese, and ground paprika.
4. Pour the mixture evenly into the muffin tin cups.
5. Bake for 20-25 minutes, or until the eggs are set.
6. Allow to cool for a few minutes before removing from the tin.
7. Serve warm.

Nutrition Info per Serving
- Calories: 90
- Protein: 7g
- Fat: 6g
- Carbohydrates: 2g
- Fiber: 1g
- Sugars: 1g

Serves
6 muffins

Cooking Time
30 minutes

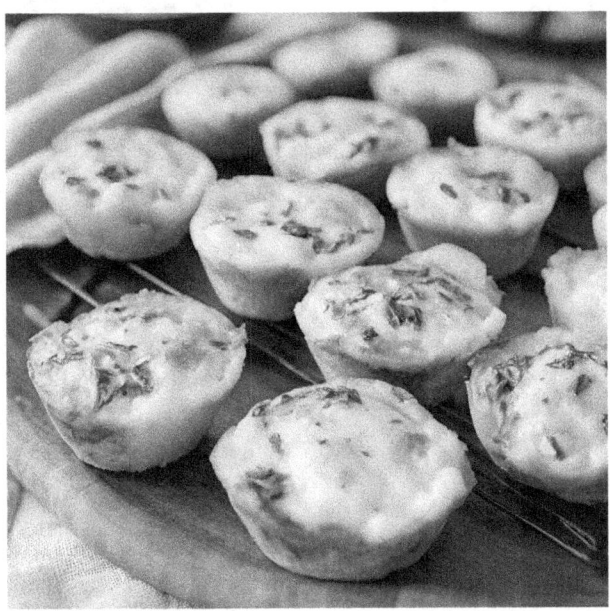

15. Soft Cheese Omelette

Ingredients
- 2 large eggs
- 2 tablespoons milk (dairy or plant-based)
- 1/4 cup soft cheese (such as ricotta or cream cheese)
- 1/4 cup chopped fresh herbs (such as chives, parsley, or basil)

Instructions
1. In a bowl, whisk together the eggs and milk.
2. Heat a non-stick skillet over medium heat.
3. Pour the egg mixture into the skillet and cook for 2-3 minutes until the edges begin to set.
4. Spread the soft cheese over one half of the omelette and sprinkle with fresh herbs.
5. Fold the omelette in half and cook for another 1-2 minutes until the cheese is melted and the eggs are fully set.
6. Serve immediately.

Nutrition Info per Serving
- Calories: 200
- Protein: 12g
- Fat: 15g
- Carbohydrates: 2g
- Fiber: 0g
- Sugars: 1g

Serves
1

Cooking Time
10 minutes

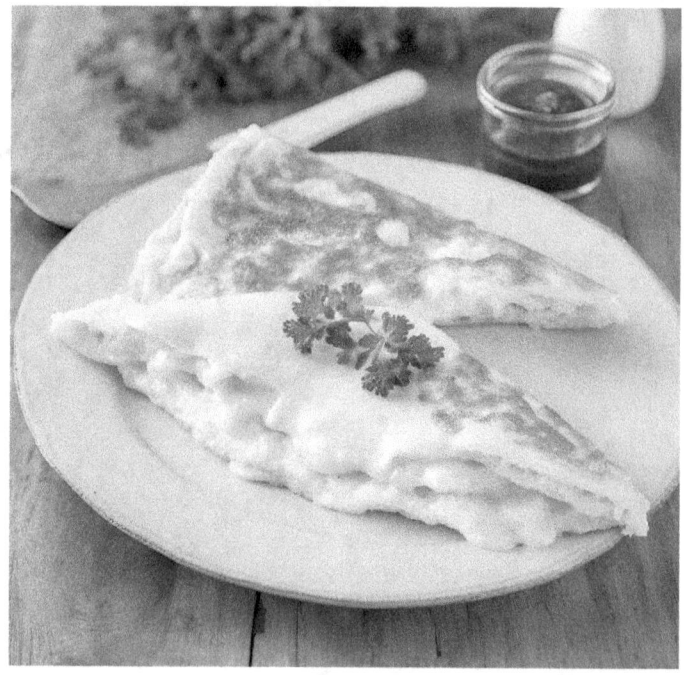

16. Peach Smoothie

Ingredients
- 1 ripe peach, pitted and sliced (or 1 cup canned peaches in juice, drained)
- 1 banana
- 1/2 cup plain Greek yogurt or plant-based yogurt
- 1/2 cup orange juice
- 1 tablespoon honey or maple syrup (optional)

Instructions
1. In a blender, combine the peach, banana, yogurt, and orange juice.
2. Blend until smooth.
3. Add honey or maple syrup if desired for sweetness.
4. Serve immediately.

Nutrition Info per Serving
- Calories: 180
- Protein: 6g
- Fat: 1g
- Carbohydrates: 40g
- Fiber: 4g
- Sugars: 30g

Serves
2

Cooking Time
5 minutes

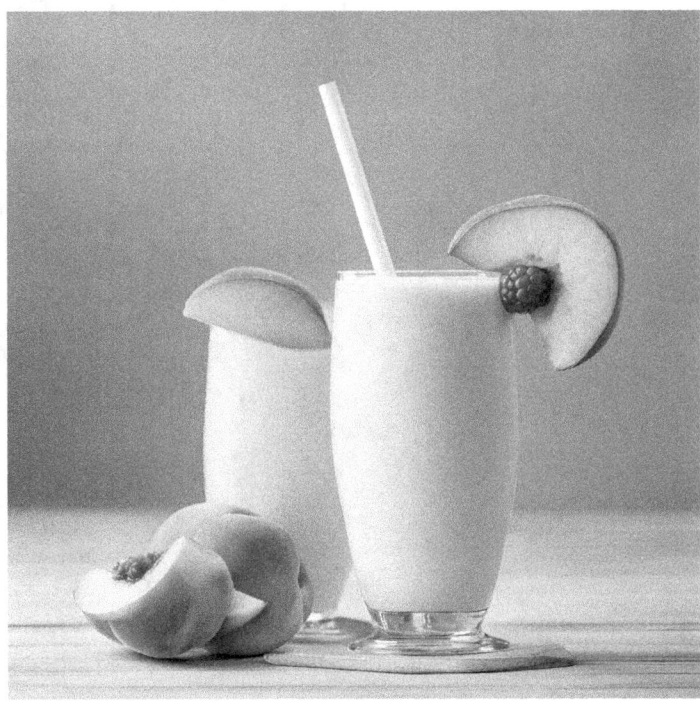

17. Cinnamon Toast

Ingredients
- 2 slices whole-grain bread
- 1 tablespoon butter or margarine
- 1 teaspoon ground cinnamon
- 1 tablespoon honey or maple syrup

Instructions
1. Toast the bread slices to your desired level of crispiness.
2. Spread the butter or margarine evenly over the toasted bread.
3. Sprinkle with ground cinnamon.
4. Drizzle with honey or maple syrup.
5. Serve immediately.

Nutrition Info per Serving
- Calories: 180
- Protein: 4g
- Fat: 7g
- Carbohydrates: 26g
- Fiber: 3g
- Sugars: 10g

Serves
1

Cooking Time
5 minutes

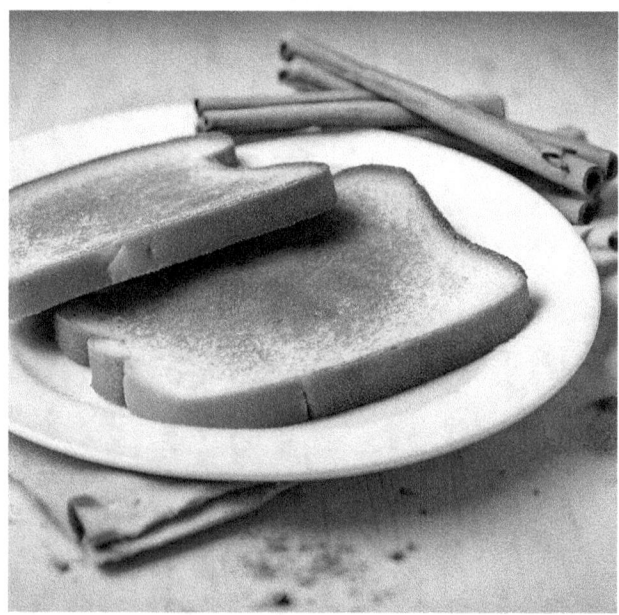

18. Baked Oatmeal
Ingredients
- 2 cups rolled oats
- 1/2 cup brown sugar
- 1 teaspoon baking powder
- 1 teaspoon ground cinnamon
- 1/2 teaspoon ground nutmeg
- 1/2 teaspoon salt
- 2 cups milk (dairy or plant-based)
- 1 large egg
- 1/4 cup melted butter or coconut oil
- 1 teaspoon vanilla extract
- 1 cup fresh or frozen berries (optional)

Instructions
1. Preheat the oven to 350°F (175°C). Grease a 9x9-inch baking dish.
2. In a large bowl, combine the oats, brown sugar, baking powder, cinnamon, nutmeg, and salt.
3. In another bowl, whisk together the milk, egg, melted butter or coconut oil, and vanilla extract.
4. Pour the wet ingredients into the dry ingredients and stir until well combined.
5. Fold in the berries if using.
6. Pour the mixture into the prepared baking dish.
7. Bake for 35-40 minutes, or until the top is golden brown and the oatmeal is set.
8. Allow to cool slightly before serving.

Nutrition Info per Serving
- Calories: 250
- Protein: 6g
- Fat: 10g
- Carbohydrates: 35g
- Fiber: 4g
- Sugars: 20g

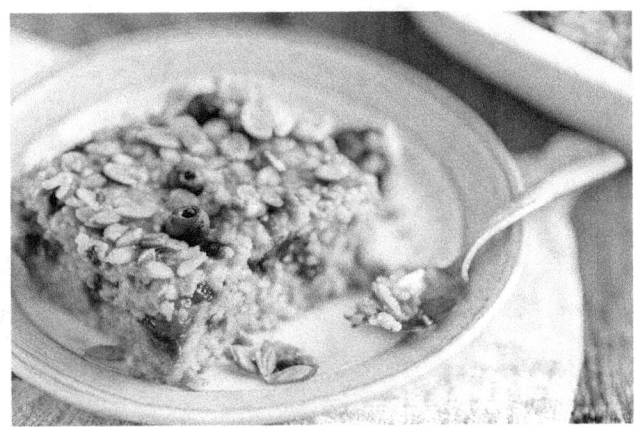

Serves
6
Cooking Time
45 minutes

19. Soft Cheese and Crackers

Ingredients

- 4 whole-grain crackers
- 1/2 cup soft cheese (such as ricotta or cream cheese)
- 1/4 cup sliced cucumber
- 1/4 cup sliced cherry tomatoes
- Optional: fresh herbs like dill or chives

Instructions

1. Spread an even layer of soft cheese on each cracker.
2. Top with sliced cucumber and cherry tomatoes.
3. Garnish with fresh herbs if desired.
4. Serve immediately.

Nutrition Info per Serving

- Calories: 150
- Protein: 5g
- Fat: 9g
- Carbohydrates: 12g
- Fiber: 2g
- Sugars: 2g

Serves

2

Cooking Time

5 minutes

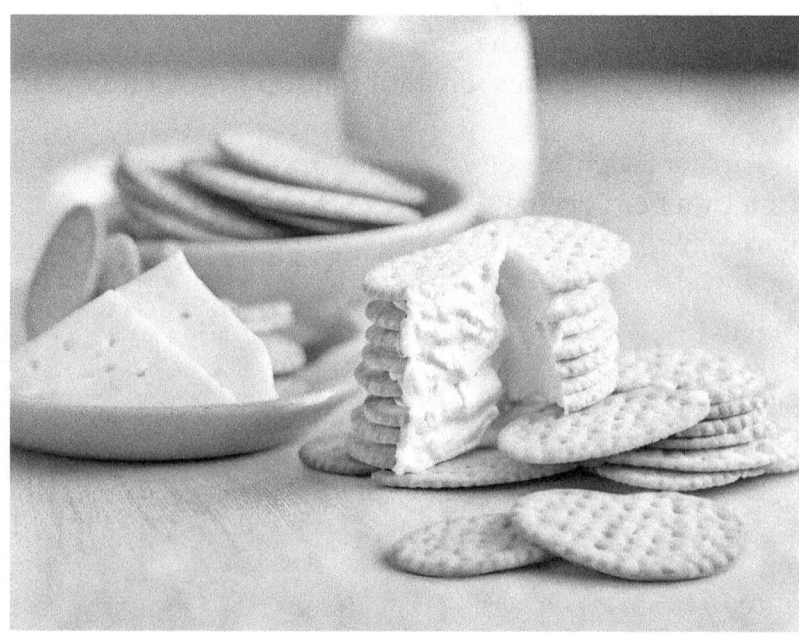

20. Egg and Cheese Quesadilla

Ingredients
- 2 large eggs
- 1/4 cup shredded cheese
- 1 whole-grain tortilla
- 1 tablespoon butter or margarine

Instructions
1. In a bowl, whisk the eggs until well beaten.
2. Heat a non-stick skillet over medium heat and add the butter or margarine.
3. Pour the eggs into the skillet and scramble until just set.
4. Remove the eggs from the skillet and set aside.
5. Place the tortilla in the skillet and sprinkle one half with shredded cheese.
6. Add the scrambled eggs on top of the cheese.
7. Fold the tortilla in half and cook until the cheese is melted and the tortilla is golden brown, about 2-3 minutes per side.
8. Remove from heat, cut into wedges, and serve immediately.

Nutrition Info per Serving
- Calories: 300
- Protein: 15g
- Fat: 18g
- Carbohydrates: 20g
- Fiber: 3g
- Sugars: 1g

Serves
1

Cooking Time
10 minutes

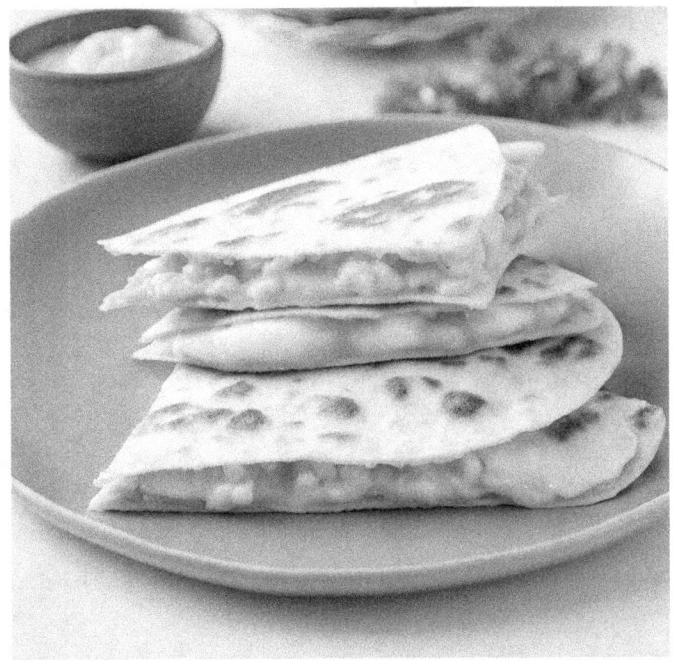

21. Creamy Semolina

Ingredients

- 1/2 cup semolina
- 2 cups milk (dairy or plant-based)
- 2 tablespoons sugar
- 1/2 teaspoon vanilla extract
- 1/4 teaspoon ground cinnamon

Instructions

1. In a medium saucepan, bring the milk to a simmer over medium heat.
2. Gradually whisk in the semolina, stirring constantly to prevent lumps.
3. Cook for 5-7 minutes, stirring frequently, until the mixture thickens.
4. Stir in the sugar, vanilla extract, and ground cinnamon.
5. Remove from heat and let it sit for a minute to thicken further.
6. Serve warm.

Nutrition Info per Serving

- Calories: 200
- Protein: 7g
- Fat: 5g
- Carbohydrates: 33g
- Fiber: 1g
- Sugars: 15g

Serves

2

Cooking Time

10 minutes

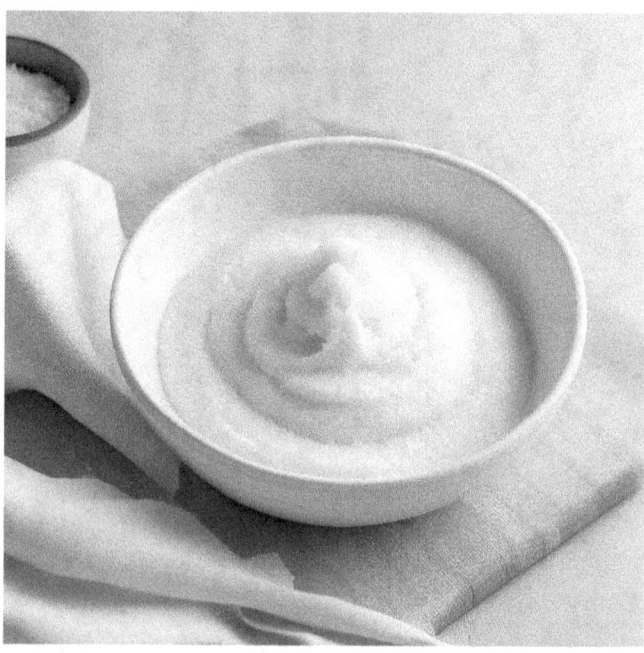

Poultry Recipes

1. Baked Chicken Breast

Ingredients
- 4 boneless, skinless chicken breasts
- 2 tablespoons olive oil
- 1 teaspoon garlic powder
- 1 teaspoon onion powder
- 1 teaspoon paprika
- 1 teaspoon dried thyme
- 1 teaspoon dried oregano
- 1/2 teaspoon ground cumin

Instructions
1. Preheat the oven to 400°F (200°C). Line a baking sheet with parchment paper.
2. In a small bowl, mix the garlic powder, onion powder, paprika, thyme, oregano, and ground cumin.
3. Rub the chicken breasts with olive oil, then sprinkle the spice mixture evenly on both sides of the chicken.
4. Place the chicken breasts on the prepared baking sheet.
5. Bake for 20-25 minutes, or until the internal temperature reaches 165°F (74°C).
6. Remove from the oven and let the chicken rest for 5 minutes before serving.

Nutrition Info per Serving
- Calories: 220
- Protein: 30g
- Fat: 10g
- Carbohydrates: 1g
- Fiber: 0g
- Sugars: 0g

Serves
4

Cooking Time
30 minutes

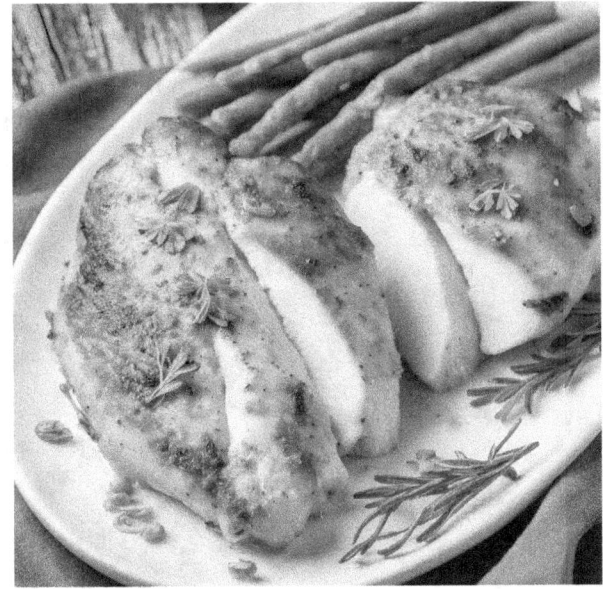

2. Chicken and Rice Soup

Ingredients
- 1 tablespoon olive oil
- 1 onion, diced
- 2 carrots, diced
- 2 celery stalks, diced
- 2 cloves garlic, minced
- 6 cups low-sodium chicken broth
- 1 cup cooked chicken breast, shredded
- 1 cup cooked brown rice
- 1 teaspoon dried thyme
- 1 teaspoon dried parsley
- 1/2 teaspoon ground turmeric

Instructions
1. Heat the olive oil in a large pot over medium heat.
2. Add the onion, carrots, and celery, and cook until softened, about 5 minutes.
3. Add the garlic and cook for another minute.
4. Pour in the chicken broth and bring to a boil.
5. Add the shredded chicken, cooked rice, thyme, parsley, and turmeric.
6. Reduce the heat and let the soup simmer for 15-20 minutes.
7. Serve hot.

Nutrition Info per Serving
- Calories: 250
- Protein: 20g
- Fat: 8g
- Carbohydrates: 25g
- Fiber: 3g
- Sugars: 4g

Serves
4

Cooking Time
30 minutes

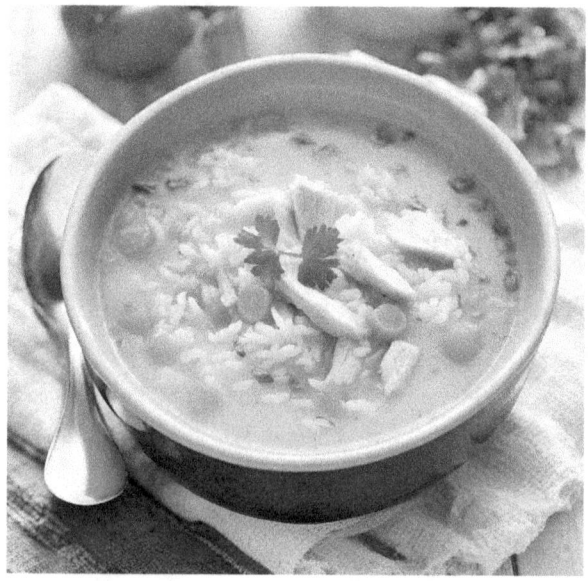

3. Chicken and Quinoa Salad

Ingredients
- 1 cup quinoa, rinsed
- 2 cups water
- 2 cups cooked chicken breast, diced
- 1 cup cherry tomatoes, halved
- 1 cucumber, diced
- 1/4 cup red onion, finely chopped
- 1/4 cup fresh parsley, chopped
- 1/4 cup olive oil
- 2 tablespoons lemon juice
- 1 teaspoon dried oregano

Instructions
1. In a medium saucepan, bring the water to a boil. Add the quinoa, reduce the heat, and simmer for 15 minutes, or until the quinoa is cooked and the water is absorbed. Let it cool.
2. In a large bowl, combine the cooked quinoa, diced chicken, cherry tomatoes, cucumber, red onion, and parsley.
3. In a small bowl, whisk together the olive oil, lemon juice, and dried oregano.
4. Pour the dressing over the salad and toss to combine.
5. Serve immediately or chill in the refrigerator until ready to serve.

Nutrition Info per Serving
- Calories: 320
- Protein: 25g
- Fat: 14g
- Carbohydrates: 25g
- Fiber: 4g
- Sugars: 3g

Serves
4

Cooking Time
25 minutes

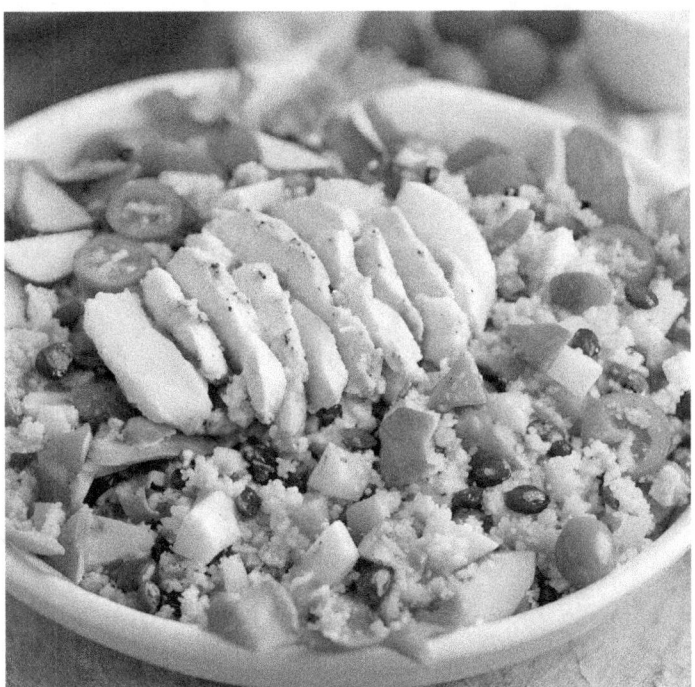

4. Poached Chicken

Ingredients
- 4 boneless, skinless chicken breasts
- 4 cups low-sodium chicken broth
- 2 cloves garlic, smashed
- 1 bay leaf
- 1 teaspoon dried thyme
- 1 teaspoon dried rosemary

Instructions
1. In a large pot, combine the chicken broth, garlic, bay leaf, thyme, and rosemary. Bring to a simmer over medium heat.
2. Add the chicken breasts to the pot. Ensure they are fully submerged in the liquid.
3. Reduce the heat to low and cover the pot. Poach the chicken for 15-20 minutes, or until the internal temperature reaches 165°F (74°C).
4. Remove the chicken from the pot and let it rest for a few minutes before slicing or shredding.
5. Serve immediately or use in other recipes.

Nutrition Info per Serving
- Calories: 180
- Protein: 30g
- Fat: 4g
- Carbohydrates: 0g
- Fiber: 0g
- Sugars: 0g

Serves
4

Cooking Time
25 minutes

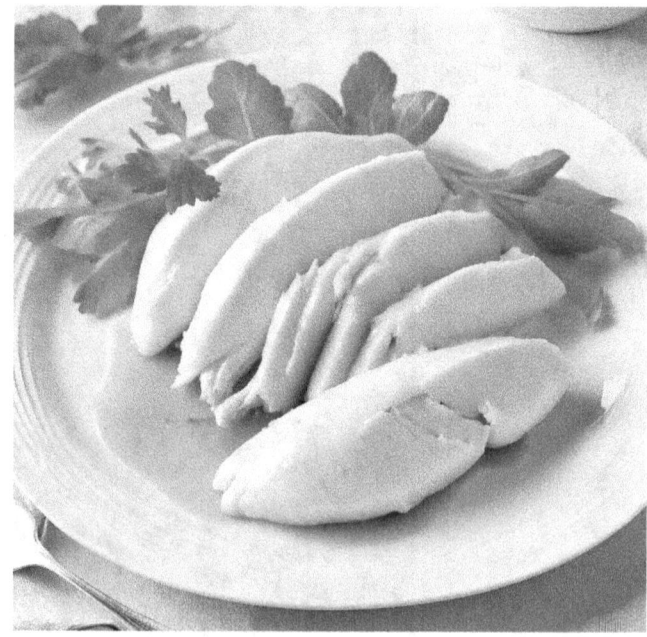

5. Lemon Herb Chicken

Ingredients
- 4 boneless, skinless chicken breasts
- 2 tablespoons olive oil
- 2 tablespoons lemon juice
- 1 tablespoon dried oregano
- 1 tablespoon dried thyme
- 2 cloves garlic, minced
- 1 lemon, sliced

Instructions
1. Preheat the oven to 375°F (190°C).
2. In a bowl, mix olive oil, lemon juice, oregano, thyme, and minced garlic.
3. Rub the chicken breasts with the mixture and place them in a baking dish.
4. Arrange lemon slices on top of the chicken.
5. Bake for 25-30 minutes, or until the internal temperature reaches 165°F (74°C).
6. Let the chicken rest for 5 minutes before serving.

Nutrition Info per Serving
- Calories: 210
- Protein: 30g
- Fat: 10g
- Carbohydrates: 2g
- Fiber: 1g
- Sugars: 0g

Serves
4

Cooking Time
35 minutes

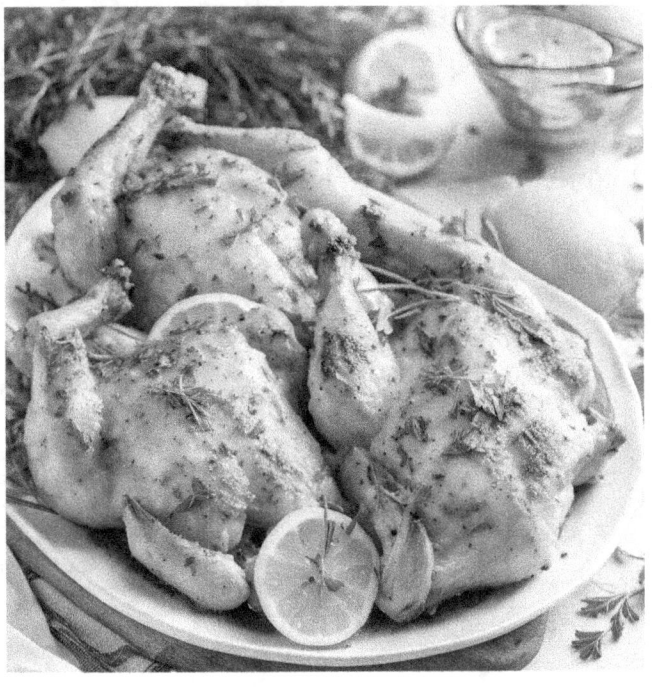

6. Chicken and Carrot Stew

Ingredients
- 2 tablespoons olive oil
- 1 onion, chopped
- 2 cloves garlic, minced
- 4 boneless, skinless chicken thighs, cut into chunks
- 4 carrots, sliced
- 4 cups low-sodium chicken broth
- 1 teaspoon dried thyme
- 1 teaspoon dried rosemary

Instructions
1. Heat olive oil in a large pot over medium heat.
2. Add onion and garlic, and sauté until soft, about 5 minutes.
3. Add chicken chunks and cook until browned, about 5 minutes.
4. Add carrots, chicken broth, thyme, and rosemary.
5. Bring to a boil, then reduce heat and simmer for 25-30 minutes, or until the chicken is cooked through and the carrots are tender.
6. Serve hot.

Nutrition Info per Serving
- Calories: 250
- Protein: 20g
- Fat: 12g
- Carbohydrates: 15g
- Fiber: 4g
- Sugars: 6g

Serves
4

Cooking Time
40 minutes

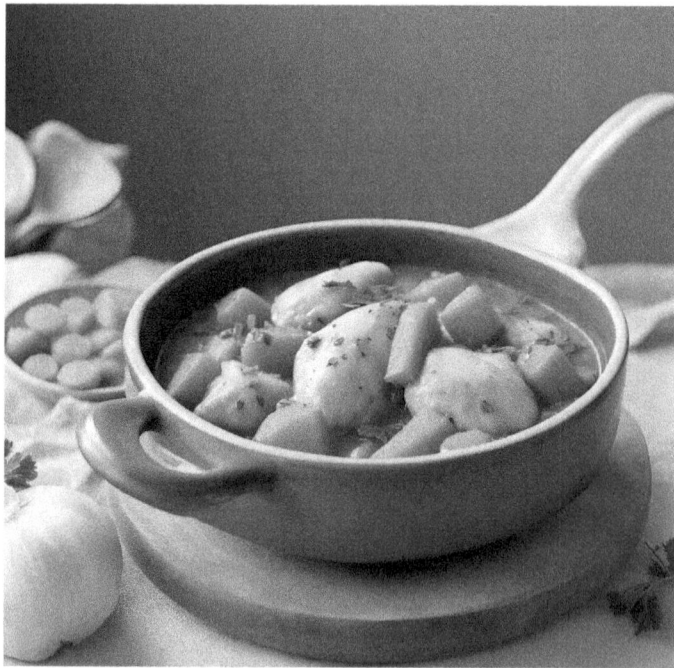

7. Chicken and Sweet Potato Bake

Ingredients
- 4 boneless, skinless chicken breasts
- 2 large sweet potatoes, peeled and cubed
- 2 tablespoons olive oil
- 1 teaspoon ground cumin
- 1 teaspoon ground paprika
- 1 teaspoon dried parsley

Instructions
1. Preheat the oven to 375°F (190°C).
2. In a large bowl, toss sweet potato cubes with olive oil, cumin, and paprika.
3. Place chicken breasts and seasoned sweet potatoes in a baking dish.
4. Sprinkle with dried parsley.
5. Bake for 30-35 minutes, or until the chicken is cooked through and the sweet potatoes are tender.
6. Let it rest for 5 minutes before serving.

Nutrition Info per Serving
- Calories: 300
- Protein: 25g
- Fat: 12g
- Carbohydrates: 25g
- Fiber: 4g
- Sugars: 8g

Serves
4

Cooking Time
40 minutes

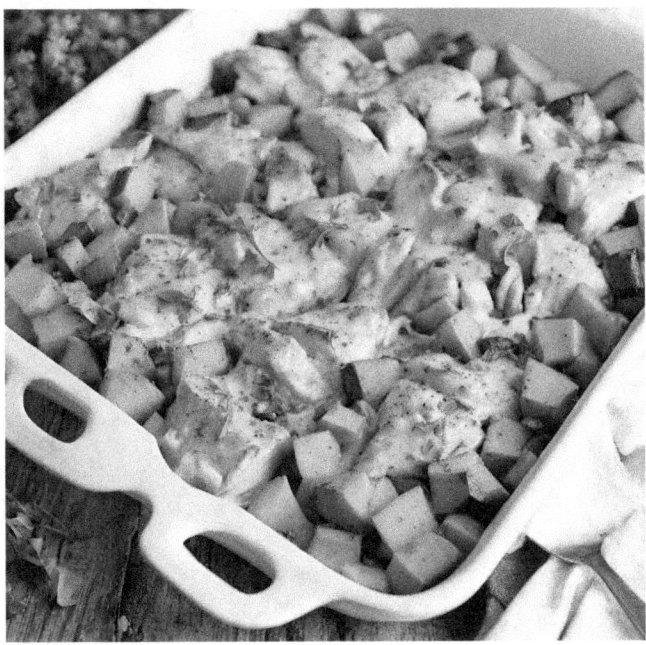

8. Chicken and Broccoli Casserole

Ingredients
- 4 boneless, skinless chicken breasts, cooked and shredded
- 4 cups broccoli florets
- 2 cups cooked brown rice
- 1 cup shredded cheddar cheese
- 1 cup plain Greek yogurt
- 1 teaspoon garlic powder
- 1 teaspoon onion powder

Instructions
1. Preheat the oven to 350°F (175°C).
2. In a large bowl, combine shredded chicken, broccoli florets, cooked rice, cheddar cheese, Greek yogurt, garlic powder, and onion powder.
3. Transfer the mixture to a greased casserole dish.
4. Bake for 25-30 minutes, or until the cheese is melted and the casserole is heated through.
5. Serve hot.

Nutrition Info per Serving
- Calories: 350
- Protein: 30g
- Fat: 15g
- Carbohydrates: 25g
- Fiber: 5g
- Sugars: 4g

Serves
6

Cooking Time
40 minutes

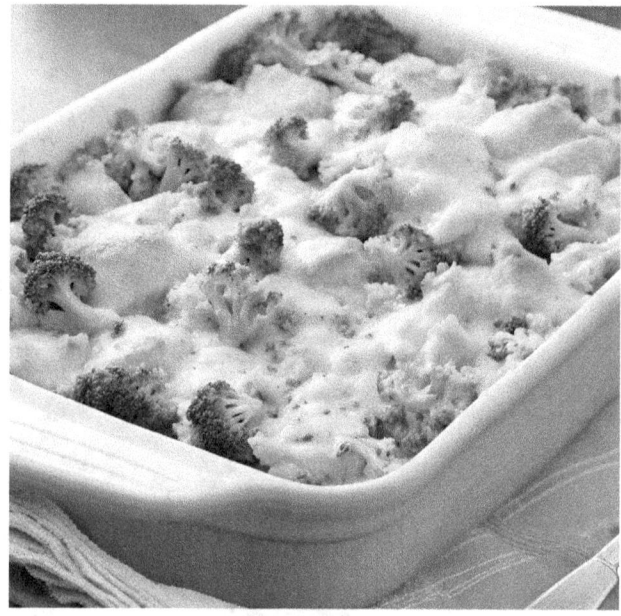

9. Chicken Meatballs

Ingredients
- 1 lb ground chicken
- 1/2 cup breadcrumbs
- 1/4 cup grated Parmesan cheese
- 1 egg
- 2 cloves garlic, minced
- 1 tablespoon dried Italian seasoning

Instructions
1. Preheat the oven to 375°F (190°C). Line a baking sheet with parchment paper.
2. In a large bowl, mix ground chicken, breadcrumbs, Parmesan cheese, egg, minced garlic, and Italian seasoning until well combined.
3. Form the mixture into small meatballs and place them on the prepared baking sheet.
4. Bake for 20-25 minutes, or until the meatballs are cooked through and golden brown.
5. Serve hot.

Nutrition Info per Serving
- Calories: 180
- Protein: 20g
- Fat: 8g
- Carbohydrates: 8g
- Fiber: 1g
- Sugars: 0g

Serves
4

Cooking Time
30 minutes

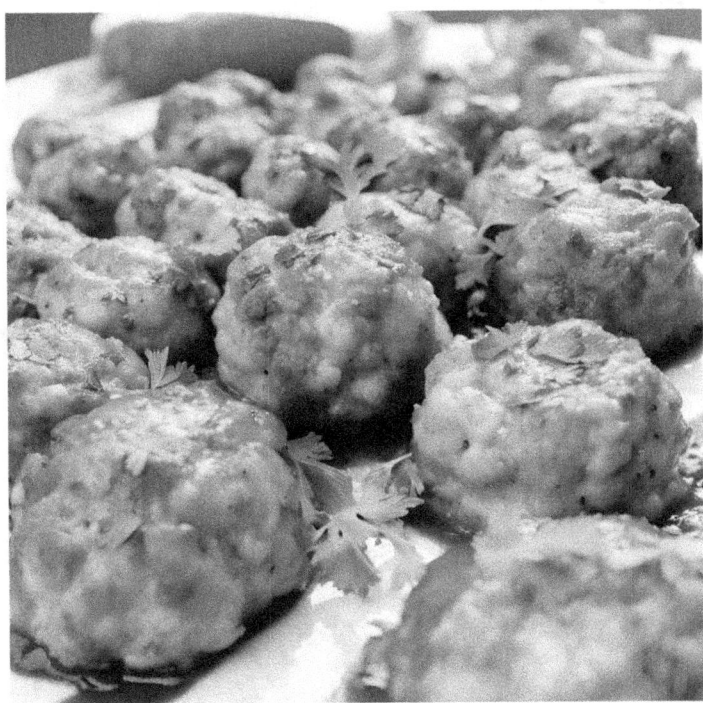

10. Chicken and Zucchini Skewers

Ingredients
- 2 boneless, skinless chicken breasts, cut into chunks
- 2 zucchinis, sliced
- 2 tablespoons olive oil
- 1 tablespoon dried oregano
- 1 tablespoon dried thyme
- 2 cloves garlic, minced

Instructions
1. Preheat the grill to medium-high heat.
2. In a bowl, mix olive oil, oregano, thyme, and minced garlic.
3. Thread chicken chunks and zucchini slices onto skewers, alternating between the two.
4. Brush the skewers with the olive oil mixture.
5. Grill the skewers for 10-12 minutes, turning occasionally, until the chicken is cooked through.
6. Serve immediately.

Nutrition Info per Serving
- Calories: 150
- Protein: 18g
- Fat: 7g
- Carbohydrates: 4g
- Fiber: 2g
- Sugars: 2g

Serves
4

Cooking Time
15 minutes

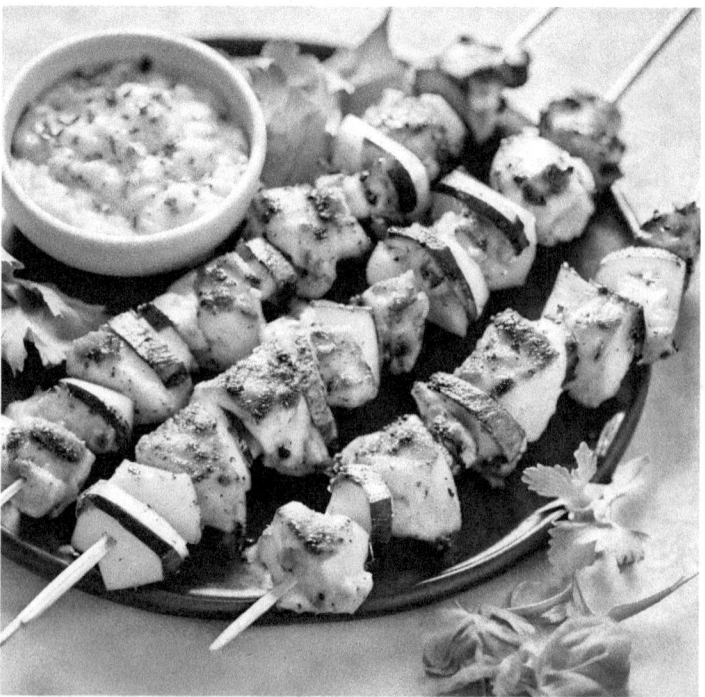

11. Chicken and Spinach Frittata

Ingredients
- 6 large eggs
- 1/2 cup milk (dairy or plant-based)
- 1 cup cooked chicken breast, shredded
- 1 cup fresh spinach, chopped
- 1/2 cup shredded mozzarella cheese
- 1 teaspoon dried basil

Instructions
1. Preheat the oven to 375°F (190°C). Grease a baking dish.
2. In a large bowl, whisk together eggs and milk.
3. Stir in shredded chicken, spinach, mozzarella cheese, and dried basil.
4. Pour the mixture into the prepared baking dish.
5. Bake for 25-30 minutes, or until the frittata is set and golden brown.
6. Let it cool for a few minutes before slicing and serving.

Nutrition Info per Serving
- Calories: 200
- Protein: 18g
- Fat: 12g
- Carbohydrates: 3g
- Fiber: 1g
- Sugars: 1g

Serves
4

Cooking Time
35 minutes

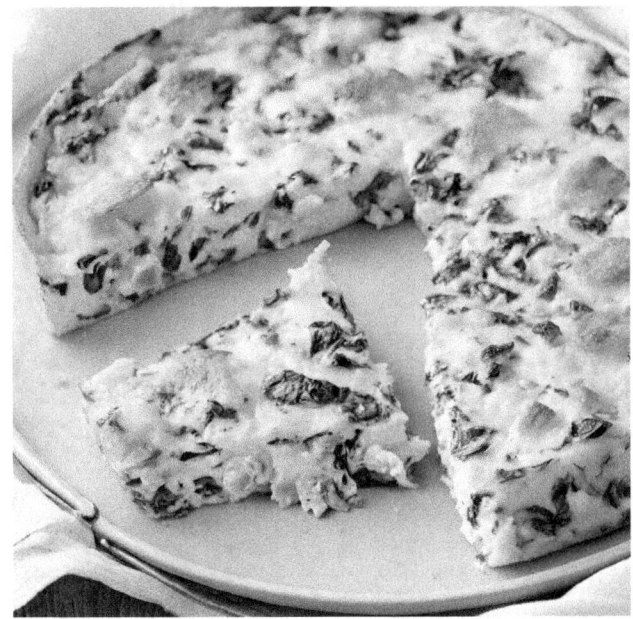

12. Chicken and Pumpkin Stew

Ingredients
- 2 tablespoons olive oil
- 1 onion, chopped
- 2 cloves garlic, minced
- 4 boneless, skinless chicken thighs, cut into chunks
- 2 cups pumpkin, peeled and cubed
- 4 cups low-sodium chicken broth
- 1 teaspoon ground cumin
- 1 teaspoon ground coriander

Instructions
1. Heat olive oil in a large pot over medium heat.
2. Add onion and garlic, and sauté until soft, about 5 minutes.
3. Add chicken chunks and cook until browned, about 5 minutes.
4. Add pumpkin cubes, chicken broth, cumin, and coriander.
5. Bring to a boil, then reduce heat and simmer for 25-30 minutes, or until the chicken is cooked through and the pumpkin is tender.
6. Serve hot.

Nutrition Info per Serving
- Calories: 260
- Protein: 20g
- Fat: 10g
- Carbohydrates: 20g
- Fiber: 4g
- Sugars: 6g

Serves
4

Cooking Time
40 minutes

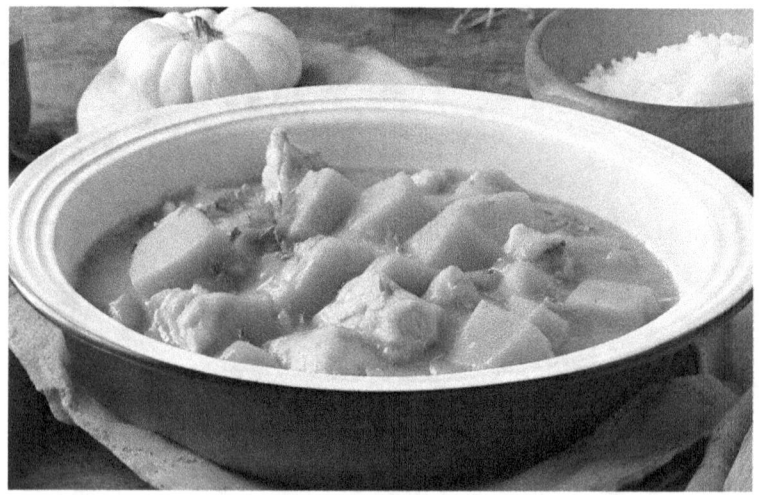

13. Chicken and Cauliflower Mash

Ingredients
- 4 boneless, skinless chicken breasts
- 1 head of cauliflower, cut into florets
- 2 tablespoons olive oil
- 1/4 cup milk (dairy or plant-based)
- 1/4 cup grated Parmesan cheese
- 1 teaspoon garlic powder

Instructions
1. Preheat the oven to 375°F (190°C).
2. Place the chicken breasts on a baking sheet and brush with 1 tablespoon of olive oil.
3. Bake for 20-25 minutes, or until the chicken is cooked through.
4. While the chicken is baking, steam the cauliflower florets until tender, about 10-15 minutes.
5. In a blender or food processor, combine the steamed cauliflower, remaining olive oil, milk, Parmesan cheese, and garlic powder. Blend until smooth.
6. Serve the baked chicken breasts with a side of cauliflower mash.

Nutrition Info per Serving
- Calories: 250
- Protein: 28g
- Fat: 12g
- Carbohydrates: 8g
- Fiber: 3g
- Sugars: 3g

Serves
4

Cooking Time
30 minutes

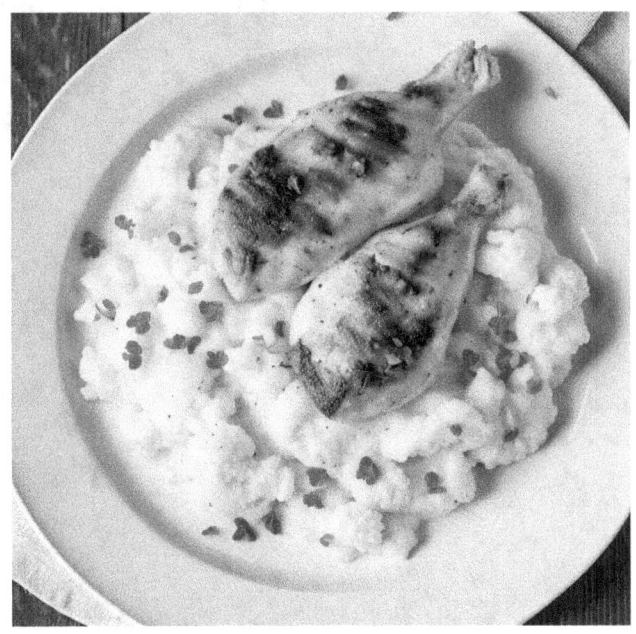

14. Chicken and Apple Salad

Ingredients
- 2 cups cooked chicken breast, diced
- 1 large apple, diced
- 1/2 cup celery, chopped
- 1/4 cup walnuts, chopped
- 1/4 cup dried cranberries
- 1/2 cup plain Greek yogurt
- 1 tablespoon honey
- 1 teaspoon lemon juice

Instructions
1. In a large bowl, combine the diced chicken, apple, celery, walnuts, and dried cranberries.
2. In a small bowl, mix the Greek yogurt, honey, and lemon juice until well combined.
3. Pour the yogurt dressing over the salad and toss to coat.
4. Serve immediately or chill in the refrigerator until ready to serve.

Nutrition Info per Serving
- Calories: 250
- Protein: 20g
- Fat: 10g
- Carbohydrates: 20g
- Fiber: 3g
- Sugars: 15g

Serves
4

Cooking Time
10 minutes

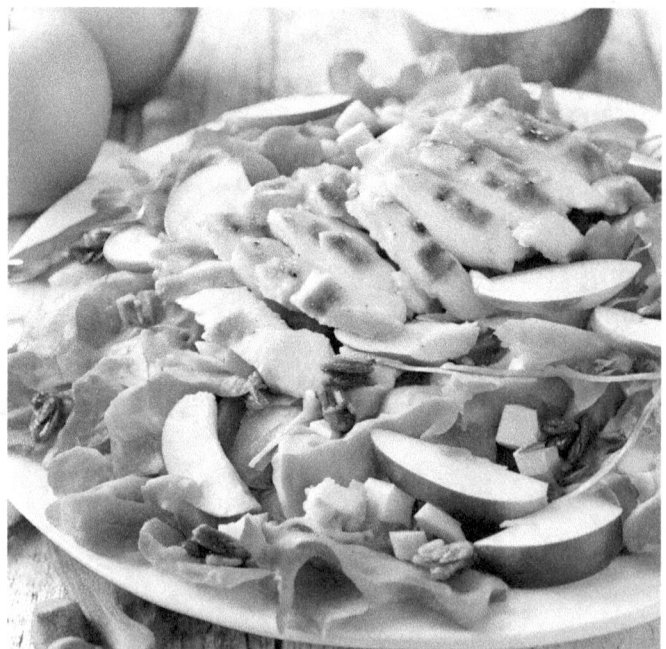

15. Chicken and Green Bean Stir-Fry

Ingredients
- 2 tablespoons vegetable oil
- 1 lb boneless, skinless chicken breasts, sliced thinly
- 2 cups green beans, trimmed
- 1 red bell pepper, sliced
- 2 cloves garlic, minced
- 1/4 cup low-sodium soy sauce
- 1 tablespoon honey
- 1 teaspoon ground ginger

Instructions
1. Heat the vegetable oil in a large skillet over medium-high heat.
2. Add the chicken slices and cook until browned, about 5 minutes.
3. Add the green beans, red bell pepper, and garlic, and stir-fry for another 3-4 minutes.
4. In a small bowl, mix the soy sauce, honey, and ground ginger.
5. Pour the sauce over the chicken and vegetables and stir to coat.
6. Cook for another 2-3 minutes, until everything is heated through.
7. Serve immediately.

Nutrition Info per Serving
- Calories: 280
- Protein: 25g
- Fat: 12g
- Carbohydrates: 15g
- Fiber: 4g
- Sugars: 10g

Serves
4

Cooking Time
20 minutes

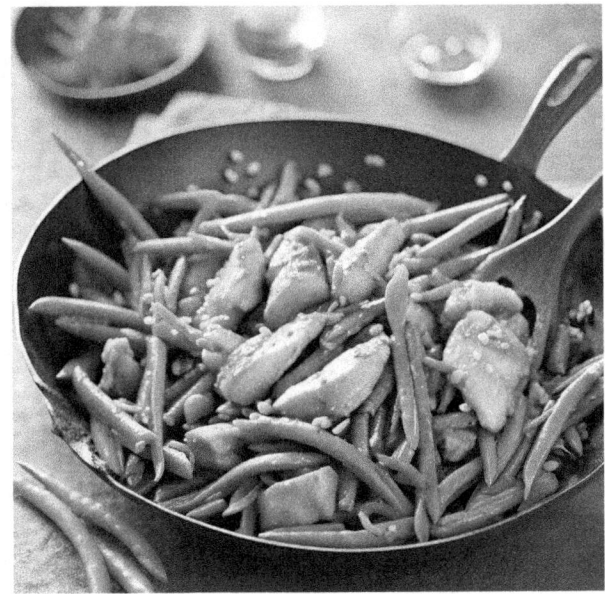

16. Chicken and Butternut Squash Bake

Ingredients
- 4 boneless, skinless chicken breasts
- 2 cups butternut squash, peeled and cubed
- 2 tablespoons olive oil
- 1 teaspoon ground cumin
- 1 teaspoon ground cinnamon
- 1/2 teaspoon dried thyme

Instructions
1. Preheat the oven to 375°F (190°C).
2. In a large bowl, toss the butternut squash cubes with olive oil, cumin, and cinnamon.
3. Place the chicken breasts and seasoned butternut squash in a baking dish.
4. Sprinkle with dried thyme.
5. Bake for 30-35 minutes, or until the chicken is cooked through and the butternut squash is tender.
6. Let it rest for 5 minutes before serving.

Nutrition Info per Serving
- Calories: 280
- Protein: 25g
- Fat: 12g
- Carbohydrates: 20g
- Fiber: 4g
- Sugars: 6g

Serves
4

Cooking Time
40 minutes

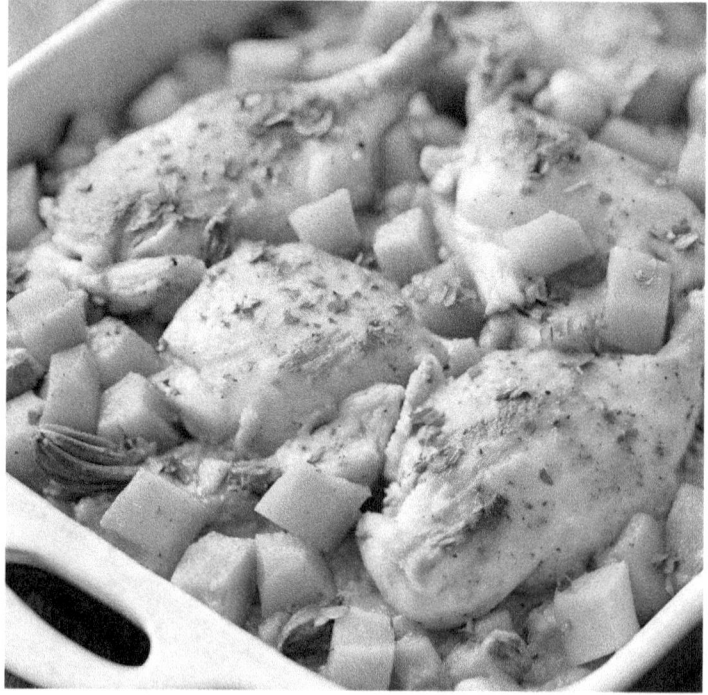

17. Chicken and Tomato Pasta

Ingredients
- 8 oz whole wheat pasta
- 1 tablespoon olive oil
- 1 lb boneless, skinless chicken breasts, diced
- 2 cloves garlic, minced
- 1 can (14.5 oz) diced tomatoes
- 1 teaspoon dried basil
- 1 teaspoon dried oregano
- 1/4 cup grated Parmesan cheese

Instructions
1. Cook the pasta according to package instructions. Drain and set aside.
2. Heat the olive oil in a large skillet over medium heat.
3. Add the diced chicken and cook until browned, about 5-7 minutes.
4. Add the garlic and cook for another minute.
5. Stir in the diced tomatoes, basil, and oregano. Simmer for 10 minutes.
6. Add the cooked pasta to the skillet and toss to combine.
7. Sprinkle with grated Parmesan cheese before serving.

Nutrition Info per Serving
- Calories: 350
- Protein: 30g
- Fat: 10g
- Carbohydrates: 35g
- Fiber: 6g
- Sugars: 6g

Serves
4

Cooking Time
30 minutes

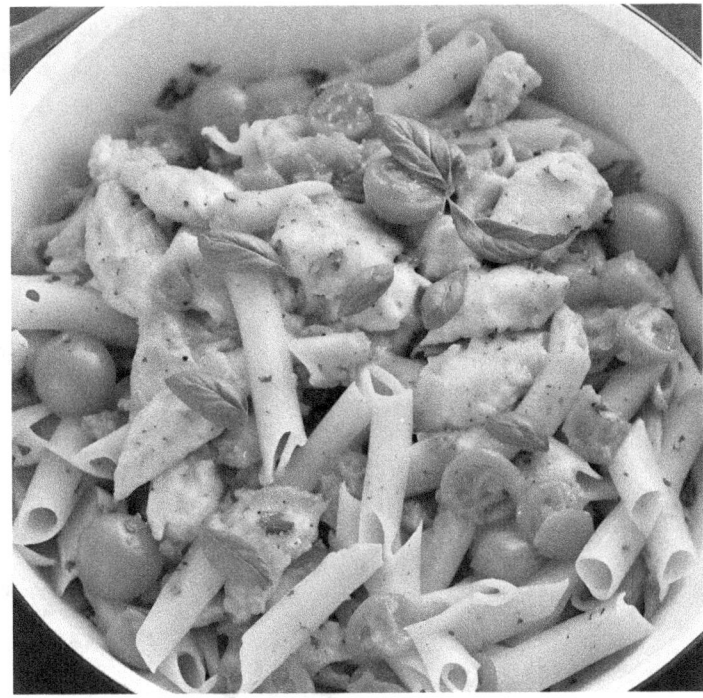

18. Chicken and Pea Risotto

Ingredients
- 1 tablespoon olive oil
- 1 onion, finely chopped
- 1 cup Arborio rice
- 4 cups low-sodium chicken broth, warmed
- 1 cup cooked chicken breast, shredded
- 1 cup frozen peas
- 1/4 cup grated Parmesan cheese
- 1 teaspoon dried thyme

Instructions
1. Heat the olive oil in a large saucepan over medium heat.
2. Add the onion and cook until soft, about 5 minutes.
3. Add the Arborio rice and cook for 2-3 minutes, stirring frequently.
4. Gradually add the warmed chicken broth, one ladle at a time, stirring constantly until each addition is absorbed before adding more.
5. Continue this process until the rice is tender and creamy, about 20 minutes.
6. Stir in the shredded chicken, peas, Parmesan cheese, and thyme.
7. Cook for another 2-3 minutes, until everything is heated through.
8. Serve immediately.

Nutrition Info per Serving
- Calories: 320
- Protein: 20g
- Fat: 10g
- Carbohydrates: 35g
- Fiber: 4g
- Sugars: 3g

Serves
4

Cooking Time
35 minutes

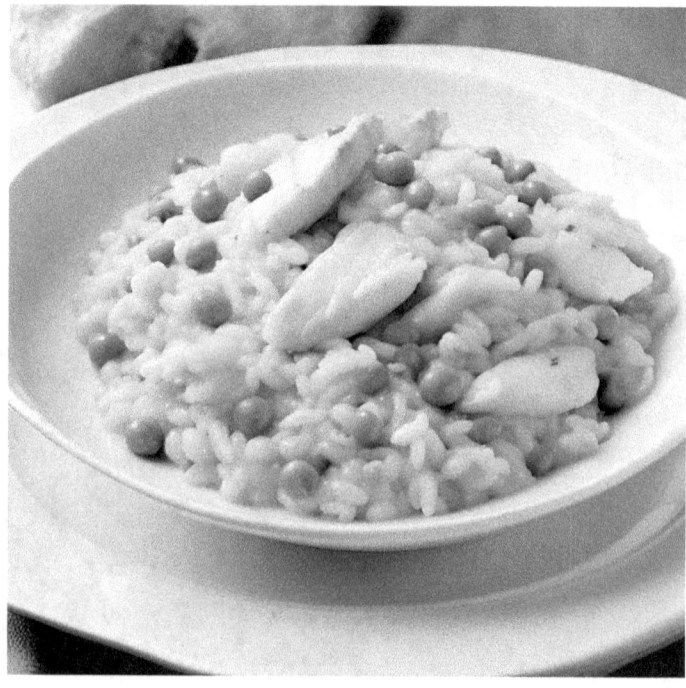

19. Chicken and Carrot Puree

Ingredients
- 2 boneless, skinless chicken breasts
- 4 large carrots, peeled and chopped
- 1 tablespoon olive oil
- 1/4 cup plain Greek yogurt
- 1 teaspoon ground cumin

Instructions
1. Preheat the oven to 375°F (190°C).
2. Place the chicken breasts on a baking sheet and brush with olive oil.
3. Bake for 20-25 minutes, or until the chicken is cooked through.
4. While the chicken is baking, steam the carrots until tender, about 10-15 minutes.
5. In a blender or food processor, combine the steamed carrots, Greek yogurt, and ground cumin. Blend until smooth.
6. Serve the baked chicken breasts with a side of carrot puree.

Nutrition Info per Serving
- Calories: 250
- Protein: 28g
- Fat: 8g
- Carbohydrates: 15g
- Fiber: 5g
- Sugars: 7g

Serves
2

Cooking Time
30 minutes

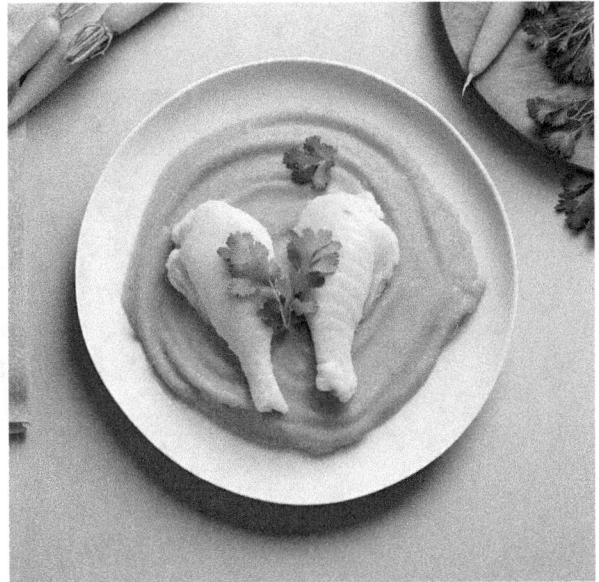

20. Chicken and Rice Paper Rolls

Ingredients
- 1 lb boneless, skinless chicken breasts, cooked and shredded
- 12 rice paper wrappers
- 1 cup shredded carrots
- 1 cup sliced cucumber
- 1/2 cup fresh mint leaves
- 1/2 cup fresh cilantro leaves
- 1/4 cup hoisin sauce for dipping

Instructions
1. Fill a shallow dish with warm water.
2. Dip one rice paper wrapper in the water for about 10 seconds to soften.
3. Lay the softened wrapper on a clean surface.
4. Place a small amount of shredded chicken, carrots, cucumber, mint, and cilantro in the center of the wrapper.
5. Fold the sides of the wrapper over the filling, then roll it up tightly.
6. Repeat with the remaining wrappers and fillings.
7. Serve the rice paper rolls with hoisin sauce for dipping.

Nutrition Info per Serving
- Calories: 150
- Protein: 18g
- Fat: 3g
- Carbohydrates: 12g
- Fiber: 2g
- Sugars: 3g

Serves
4

Cooking Time
20 minutes

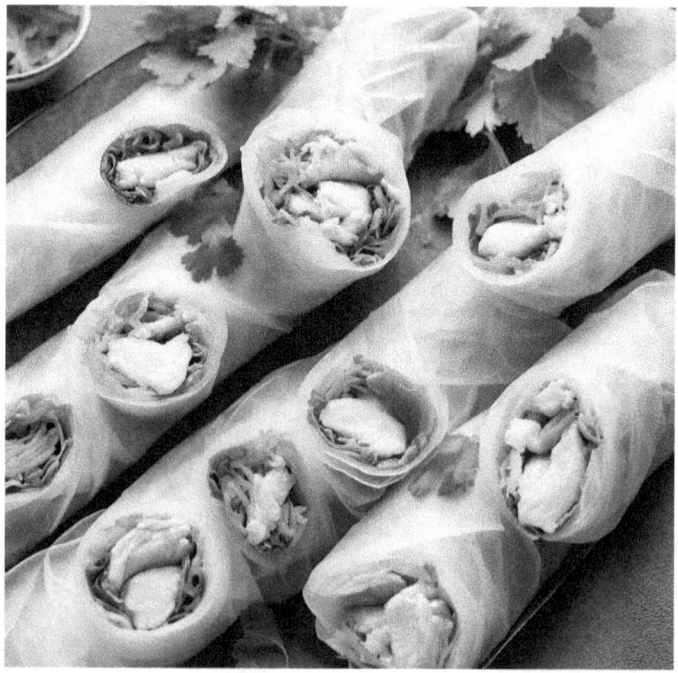

21. Chicken and Spinach Soup

Ingredients
- 1 tablespoon olive oil
- 1 onion, chopped
- 2 cloves garlic, minced
- 4 cups low-sodium chicken broth
- 2 cups cooked chicken breast, shredded
- 2 cups fresh spinach, chopped
- 1 teaspoon dried thyme

Instructions
1. Heat the olive oil in a large pot over medium heat.
2. Add the onion and garlic, and cook until soft, about 5 minutes.
3. Pour in the chicken broth and bring to a boil.
4. Add the shredded chicken, chopped spinach, and thyme.
5. Reduce the heat and simmer for 10 minutes.
6. Serve hot.

Nutrition Info per Serving
- Calories: 180
- Protein: 20g
- Fat: 8g
- Carbohydrates: 8g
- Fiber: 2g
- Sugars: 3g

Serves
4

Cooking Time
20 minutes

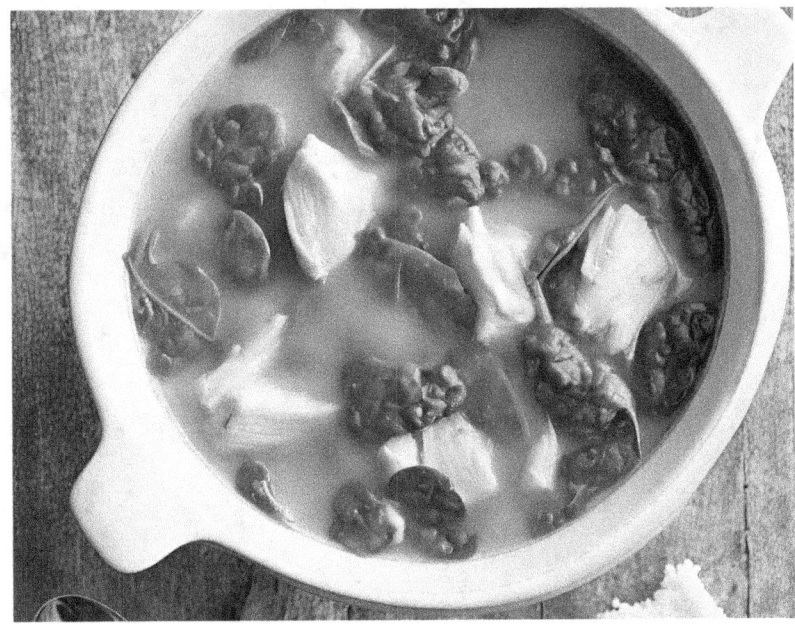

22. Chicken and Mashed Potatoes

Ingredients
- 4 boneless, skinless chicken breasts
- 1 tablespoon olive oil
- 4 large potatoes, peeled and cubed
- 1/2 cup milk (dairy or plant-based)
- 1/4 cup butter
- 1 teaspoon garlic powder

Instructions
1. Preheat the oven to 375°F (190°C).
2. Place the chicken breasts on a baking sheet and brush with olive oil.
3. Bake for 20-25 minutes, or until the chicken is cooked through.
4. While the chicken is baking, boil the potatoes in a large pot of water until tender, about 15 minutes.
5. Drain the potatoes and return them to the pot.
6. Add the milk, butter, and garlic powder to the potatoes. Mash until smooth.
7. Serve the baked chicken breasts with a side of mashed potatoes.

Nutrition Info per Serving
- Calories: 300
- Protein: 30g
- Fat: 12g
- Carbohydrates: 20g
- Fiber: 3g
- Sugars: 2g

Serves
4

Cooking Time
30 minutes

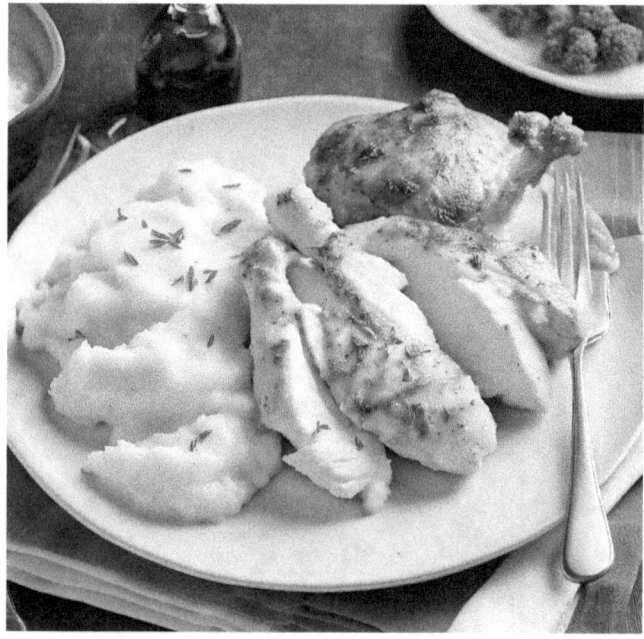

23. Baked Turkey Breast

Ingredients
- 2 lbs boneless turkey breast
- 2 tablespoons olive oil
- 1 teaspoon garlic powder
- 1 teaspoon dried thyme
- 1 teaspoon dried rosemary
- 1/2 teaspoon paprika

Instructions
1. Preheat the oven to 375°F (190°C).
2. In a small bowl, mix the olive oil, garlic powder, thyme, rosemary, and paprika.
3. Rub the turkey breast with the olive oil mixture and place it in a baking dish.
4. Bake for 45-55 minutes, or until the internal temperature reaches 165°F (74°C).
5. Let the turkey rest for 10 minutes before slicing.
6. Serve warm.

Nutrition Info per Serving
- Calories: 220
- Protein: 35g
- Fat: 10g
- Carbohydrates: 1g
- Fiber: 0g
- Sugars: 0g

Serves
4

Cooking Time
55 minutes

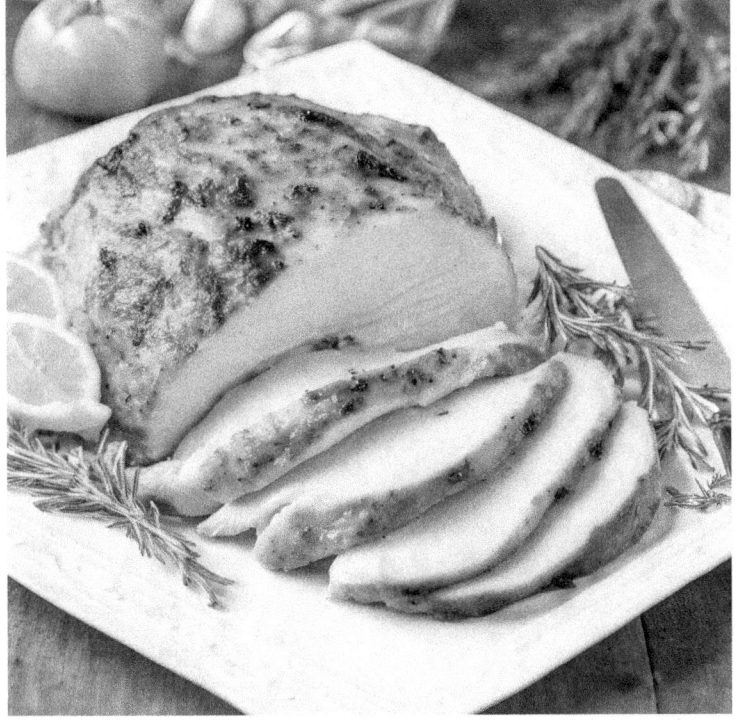

24. Turkey and Vegetable Soup

Ingredients

- 1 tablespoon olive oil
- 1 onion, chopped
- 2 cloves garlic, minced
- 2 cups cooked turkey breast, shredded
- 2 carrots, sliced
- 2 celery stalks, sliced
- 4 cups low-sodium turkey or chicken broth
- 1 teaspoon dried thyme
- 1 teaspoon dried parsley

Instructions

1. Heat the olive oil in a large pot over medium heat.
2. Add the onion and garlic, and cook until soft, about 5 minutes.
3. Add the shredded turkey, carrots, and celery.
4. Pour in the broth and bring to a boil.
5. Add the thyme and parsley, then reduce the heat and simmer for 20 minutes.
6. Serve hot.

Nutrition Info per Serving

- Calories: 180
- Protein: 20g
- Fat: 7g
- Carbohydrates: 8g
- Fiber: 2g
- Sugars: 3g

Serves

4

Cooking Time

30 minutes

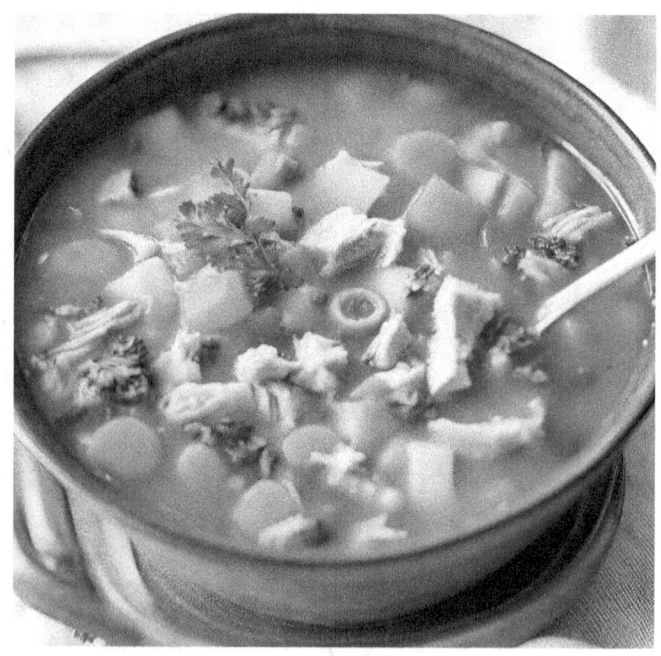

25. Turkey and Quinoa Salad

Ingredients
- 1 cup quinoa, rinsed
- 2 cups water
- 2 cups cooked turkey breast, diced
- 1 cup cherry tomatoes, halved
- 1 cucumber, diced
- 1/4 cup red onion, finely chopped
- 1/4 cup fresh parsley, chopped
- 1/4 cup olive oil
- 2 tablespoons lemon juice
- 1 teaspoon dried oregano

Instructions
1. In a medium saucepan, bring the water to a boil. Add the quinoa, reduce the heat, and simmer for 15 minutes, or until the quinoa is cooked and the water is absorbed. Let it cool.
2. In a large bowl, combine the cooked quinoa, diced turkey, cherry tomatoes, cucumber, red onion, and parsley.
3. In a small bowl, whisk together the olive oil, lemon juice, and oregano.
4. Pour the dressing over the salad and toss to combine.
5. Serve immediately or chill in the refrigerator until ready to serve.

Nutrition Info per Serving
- Calories: 320
- Protein: 25g
- Fat: 14g
- Carbohydrates: 25g
- Fiber: 4g
- Sugars: 3g

Serves
4

Cooking Time
25 minutes

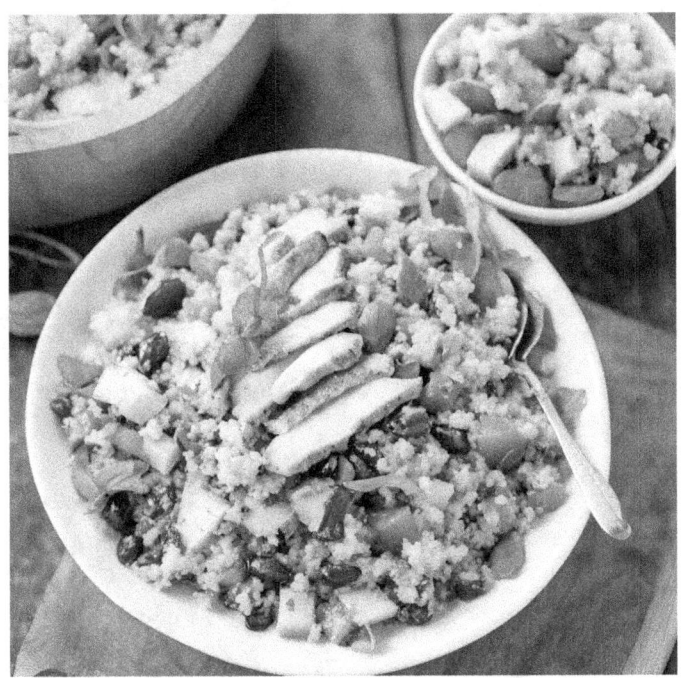

26. Turkey and Sweet Potato Hash

Ingredients
- 1 tablespoon olive oil
- 1 onion, chopped
- 2 cups cooked turkey breast, diced
- 2 large sweet potatoes, peeled and cubed
- 1 teaspoon ground cumin
- 1 teaspoon ground paprika
- 1/2 teaspoon dried thyme

Instructions
1. Heat the olive oil in a large skillet over medium heat.
2. Add the onion and cook until soft, about 5 minutes.
3. Add the diced turkey and sweet potatoes.
4. Sprinkle with cumin, paprika, and thyme.
5. Cook, stirring occasionally, for 15-20 minutes, or until the sweet potatoes are tender and slightly crispy.
6. Serve hot.

Nutrition Info per Serving
- Calories: 250
- Protein: 25g
- Fat: 8g
- Carbohydrates: 25g
- Fiber: 4g
- Sugars: 6g

Serves
4

Cooking Time
30 minutes

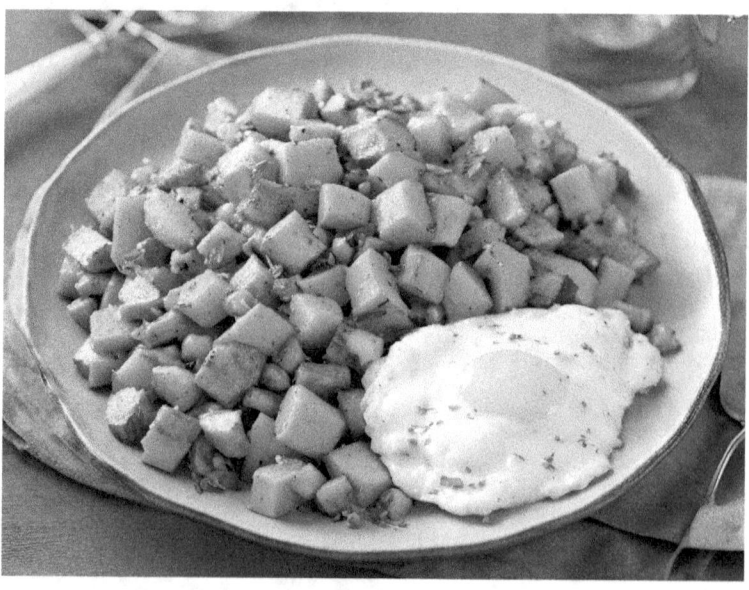

27. Turkey Meatballs

Ingredients
- 1 lb ground turkey
- 1/2 cup breadcrumbs
- 1/4 cup grated Parmesan cheese
- 1 egg
- 2 cloves garlic, minced
- 1 tablespoon dried Italian seasoning

Instructions
1. Preheat the oven to 375°F (190°C). Line a baking sheet with parchment paper.
2. In a large bowl, mix ground turkey, breadcrumbs, Parmesan cheese, egg, minced garlic, and Italian seasoning until well combined.
3. Form the mixture into small meatballs and place them on the prepared baking sheet.
4. Bake for 20-25 minutes, or until the meatballs are cooked through and golden brown.
5. Serve hot.

Nutrition Info per Serving
- Calories: 180
- Protein: 20g
- Fat: 8g
- Carbohydrates: 8g
- Fiber: 1g
- Sugars: 0g

Serves
4

Cooking Time
30 minutes

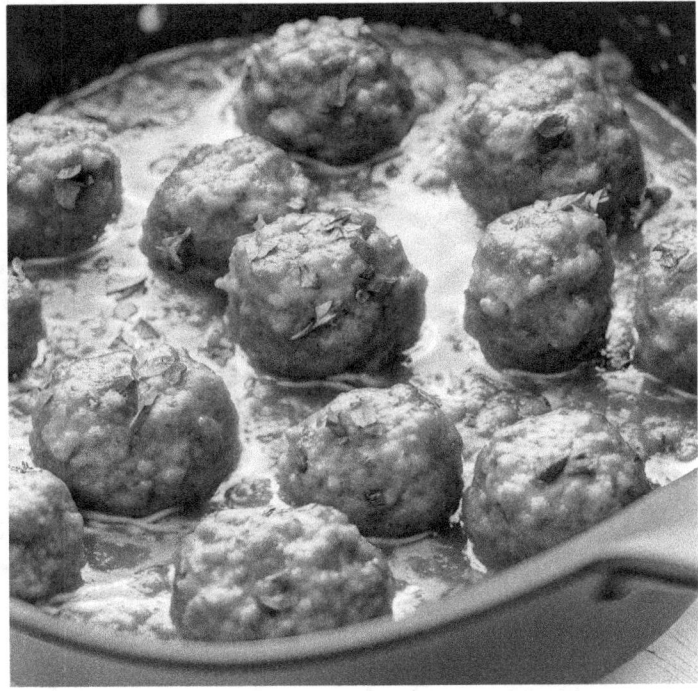

Beef and Pork Recipes

1. Beef and Rice Soup
Ingredients
- 1 tablespoon olive oil
- 1 onion, chopped
- 2 cloves garlic, minced
- 1 lb lean ground beef
- 4 cups low-sodium beef broth
- 1 cup cooked brown rice
- 2 carrots, sliced
- 2 celery stalks, sliced
- 1 teaspoon dried thyme
- 1 teaspoon dried oregano

Instructions
1. Heat the olive oil in a large pot over medium heat.
2. Add the onion and garlic, and cook until soft, about 5 minutes.
3. Add the ground beef and cook until browned, about 5-7 minutes.
4. Stir in the beef broth, cooked rice, carrots, celery, thyme, and oregano.
5. Bring to a boil, then reduce heat and simmer for 20 minutes.
6. Serve hot.

Nutrition Info per Serving
- Calories: 300
- Protein: 20g
- Fat: 12g
- Carbohydrates: 25g
- Fiber: 4g
- Sugars: 3g

Serves
4

Cooking Time
30 minutes

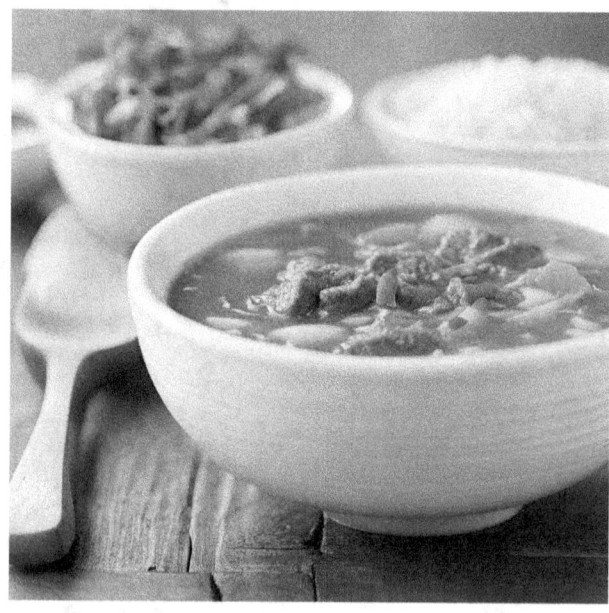

2. Beef Stew

Ingredients
- 2 tablespoons olive oil
- 1 lb beef stew meat, cubed
- 1 onion, chopped
- 2 cloves garlic, minced
- 4 cups low-sodium beef broth
- 2 potatoes, peeled and cubed
- 2 carrots, sliced
- 2 celery stalks, sliced
- 1 teaspoon dried thyme
- 1 teaspoon dried rosemary

Instructions
1. Heat 1 tablespoon of olive oil in a large pot over medium-high heat.
2. Add the beef and cook until browned on all sides, about 5 minutes. Remove the beef and set aside.
3. Add the remaining olive oil to the pot. Add the onion and garlic, and cook until soft, about 5 minutes.
4. Return the beef to the pot. Add the beef broth, potatoes, carrots, celery, thyme, and rosemary.
5. Bring to a boil, then reduce heat and simmer for 1 hour, or until the beef is tender.
6. Serve hot.

Nutrition Info per Serving
- Calories: 350
- Protein: 25g
- Fat: 15g
- Carbohydrates: 30g
- Fiber: 5g
- Sugars: 5g

Serves
4

Cooking Time
1 hour 20 minutes

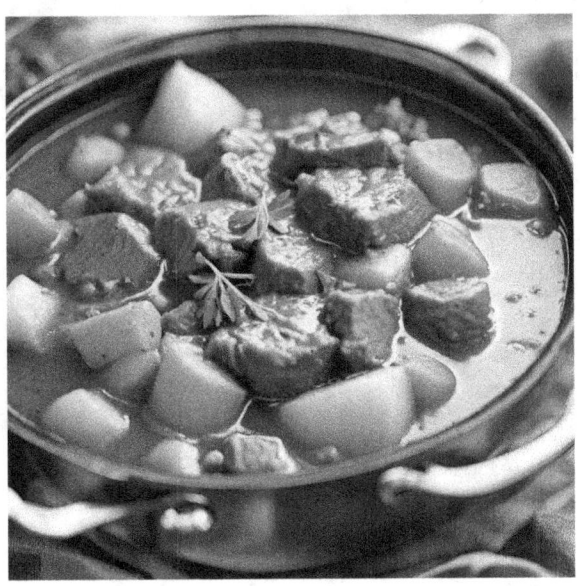

3. Ground Beef and Quinoa Bowl

Ingredients
- 1 cup quinoa, rinsed
- 2 cups water
- 1 lb lean ground beef
- 1 onion, chopped
- 1 red bell pepper, chopped
- 2 cloves garlic, minced
- 1 teaspoon ground cumin
- 1 teaspoon ground paprika
- 1/4 cup chopped fresh cilantro

Instructions
1. In a medium saucepan, bring the water to a boil. Add the quinoa, reduce heat, and simmer for 15 minutes, or until the quinoa is cooked and the water is absorbed. Let it cool.
2. In a large skillet, cook the ground beef, onion, and red bell pepper over medium heat until the beef is browned and the vegetables are soft, about 10 minutes.
3. Add the garlic, cumin, and paprika, and cook for another 2-3 minutes.
4. Stir in the cooked quinoa and cilantro.
5. Serve hot.

Nutrition Info per Serving
- Calories: 350
- Protein: 25g
- Fat: 15g
- Carbohydrates: 25g
- Fiber: 5g
- Sugars: 3g

Serves
4

Cooking Time
30 minutes

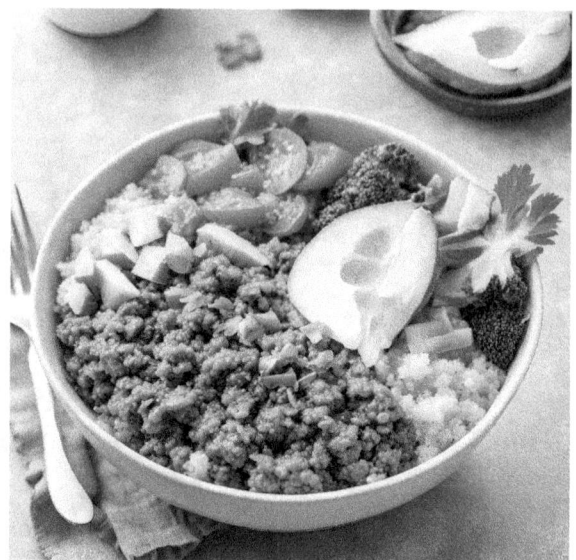

4. Beef Meatballs

Ingredients
- 1 lb lean ground beef
- 1/2 cup breadcrumbs
- 1/4 cup grated Parmesan cheese
- 1 egg
- 2 cloves garlic, minced
- 1 tablespoon dried Italian seasoning

Instructions
1. Preheat the oven to 375°F (190°C). Line a baking sheet with parchment paper.
2. In a large bowl, mix ground beef, breadcrumbs, Parmesan cheese, egg, minced garlic, and Italian seasoning until well combined.
3. Form the mixture into small meatballs and place them on the prepared baking sheet.
4. Bake for 20-25 minutes, or until the meatballs are cooked through and golden brown.
5. Serve hot.

Nutrition Info per Serving
- Calories: 200
- Protein: 22g
- Fat: 10g
- Carbohydrates: 5g
- Fiber: 1g
- Sugars: 1g

Serves
4

Cooking Time
30 minutes

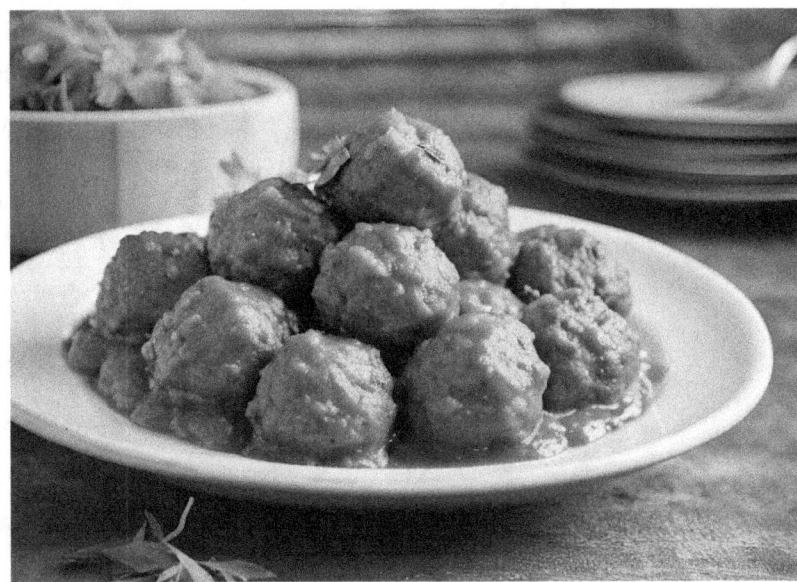

5. Pork and Rice Soup

Ingredients
- 1 tablespoon olive oil
- 1 onion, chopped
- 2 cloves garlic, minced
- 1 lb lean ground pork
- 4 cups low-sodium chicken broth
- 1 cup cooked brown rice
- 2 carrots, sliced
- 2 celery stalks, sliced
- 1 teaspoon dried thyme
- 1 teaspoon dried oregano

Instructions
1. Heat the olive oil in a large pot over medium heat.
2. Add the onion and garlic, and cook until soft, about 5 minutes.
3. Add the ground pork and cook until browned, about 5-7 minutes.
4. Stir in the chicken broth, cooked rice, carrots, celery, thyme, and oregano.
5. Bring to a boil, then reduce heat and simmer for 20 minutes.
6. Serve hot.

Nutrition Info per Serving
- Calories: 300
- Protein: 20g
- Fat: 12g
- Carbohydrates: 25g
- Fiber: 4g
- Sugars: 3g

Serves
4

Cooking Time
30 minutes

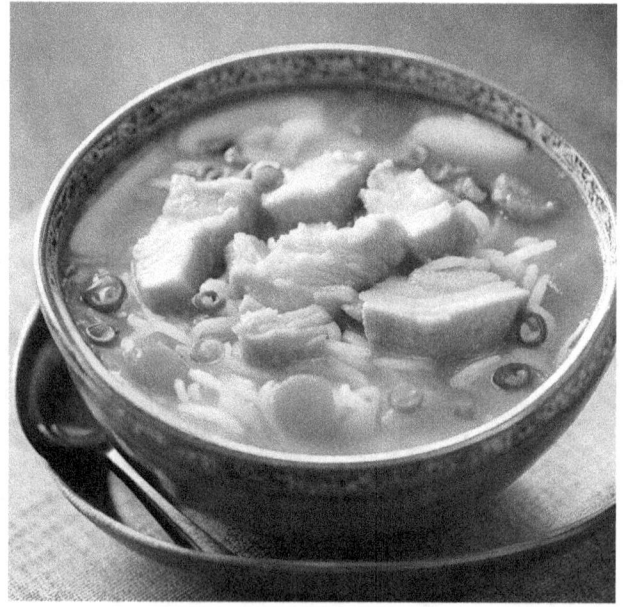

6. Pork Stew
Ingredients
- 2 tablespoons olive oil
- 1 lb pork shoulder, cubed
- 1 onion, chopped
- 2 cloves garlic, minced
- 4 cups low-sodium chicken broth
- 2 potatoes, peeled and cubed
- 2 carrots, sliced
- 2 celery stalks, sliced
- 1 teaspoon dried thyme
- 1 teaspoon dried rosemary

Instructions
1. Heat 1 tablespoon of olive oil in a large pot over medium-high heat.
2. Add the pork and cook until browned on all sides, about 5 minutes. Remove the pork and set aside.
3. Add the remaining olive oil to the pot. Add the onion and garlic, and cook until soft, about 5 minutes.
4. Return the pork to the pot. Add the chicken broth, potatoes, carrots, celery, thyme, and rosemary.
5. Bring to a boil, then reduce heat and simmer for 1 hour, or until the pork is tender.
6. Serve hot.

Nutrition Info per Serving
- Calories: 350
- Protein: 25g
- Fat: 15g
- Carbohydrates: 30g
- Fiber: 5g
- Sugars: 5g

Serves
4

Cooking Time
1 hour 20 minutes

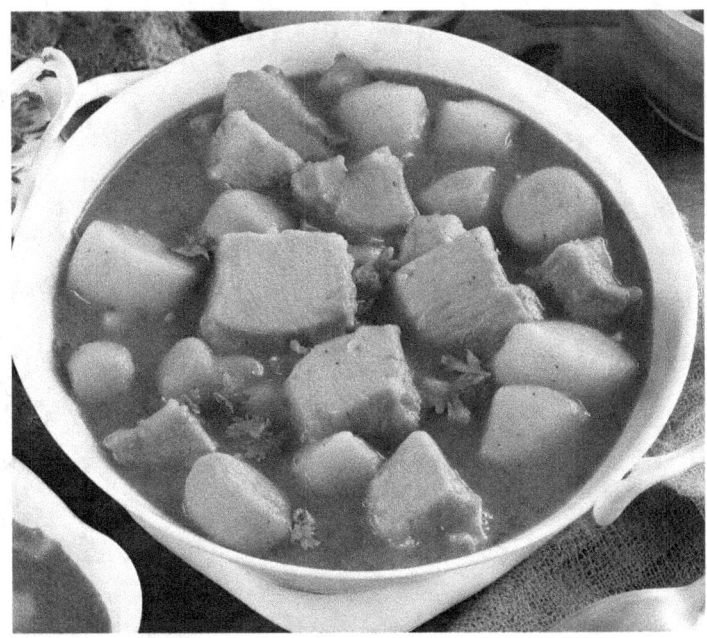

7. Pork Meatballs

Ingredients
- 1 lb lean ground pork
- 1/2 cup breadcrumbs
- 1/4 cup grated Parmesan cheese
- 1 egg
- 2 cloves garlic, minced
- 1 tablespoon dried Italian seasoning

Instructions
1. Preheat the oven to 375°F (190°C). Line a baking sheet with parchment paper.
2. In a large bowl, mix ground pork, breadcrumbs, Parmesan cheese, egg, minced garlic, and Italian seasoning until well combined.
3. Form the mixture into small meatballs and place them on the prepared baking sheet.
4. Bake for 20-25 minutes, or until the meatballs are cooked through and golden brown.
5. Serve hot.

Nutrition Info per Serving
- Calories: 200
- Protein: 22g
- Fat: 10g
- Carbohydrates: 5g
- Fiber: 1g
- Sugars: 1g

Serves
4

Cooking Time
30 minutes

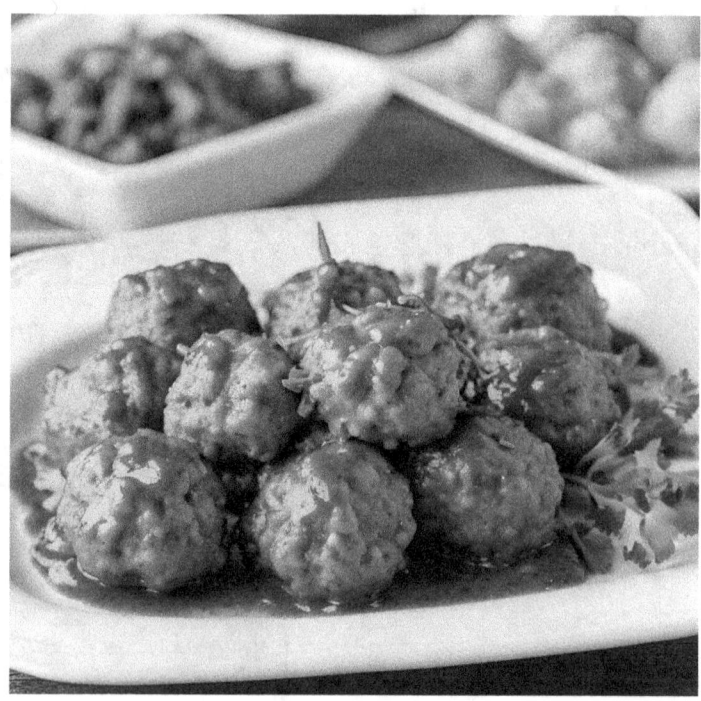

8. Pork and Apricot Salad

Ingredients
- 2 cups cooked pork tenderloin, sliced
- 1 cup dried apricots, chopped
- 1/2 cup celery, chopped
- 1/4 cup walnuts, chopped
- 1/4 cup plain Greek yogurt
- 1 tablespoon honey
- 1 teaspoon lemon juice

Instructions
1. In a large bowl, combine the sliced pork, apricots, celery, and walnuts.
2. In a small bowl, mix the Greek yogurt, honey, and lemon juice until well combined.
3. Pour the yogurt dressing over the salad and toss to coat.
4. Serve immediately or chill in the refrigerator until ready to serve.

Nutrition Info per Serving
- Calories: 250
- Protein: 20g
- Fat: 10g
- Carbohydrates: 20g
- Fiber: 3g
- Sugars: 15g

Serves
4

Cooking Time
10 minutes

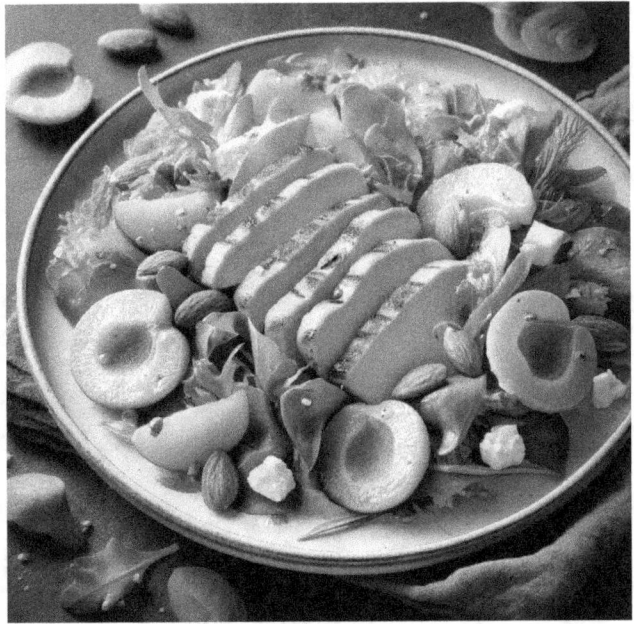

9. Pork and Vegetable Bake

Ingredients
- 4 boneless pork chops
- 2 tablespoons olive oil
- 2 cups broccoli florets
- 2 cups cauliflower florets
- 1 red bell pepper, sliced
- 1 teaspoon dried basil
- 1 teaspoon dried oregano

Instructions
1. Preheat the oven to 375°F (190°C).
2. Place the pork chops in a baking dish and brush with 1 tablespoon of olive oil.
3. In a large bowl, toss the broccoli, cauliflower, and red bell pepper with the remaining olive oil, basil, and oregano.
4. Arrange the vegetables around the pork chops in the baking dish.
5. Bake for 25-30 minutes, or until the pork is cooked through and the vegetables are tender.
6. Let it rest for 5 minutes before serving.

Nutrition Info per Serving
- Calories: 300
- Protein: 25g
- Fat: 15g
- Carbohydrates: 15g
- Fiber: 5g
- Sugars: 5g

Serves
4

Cooking Time
35 minutes

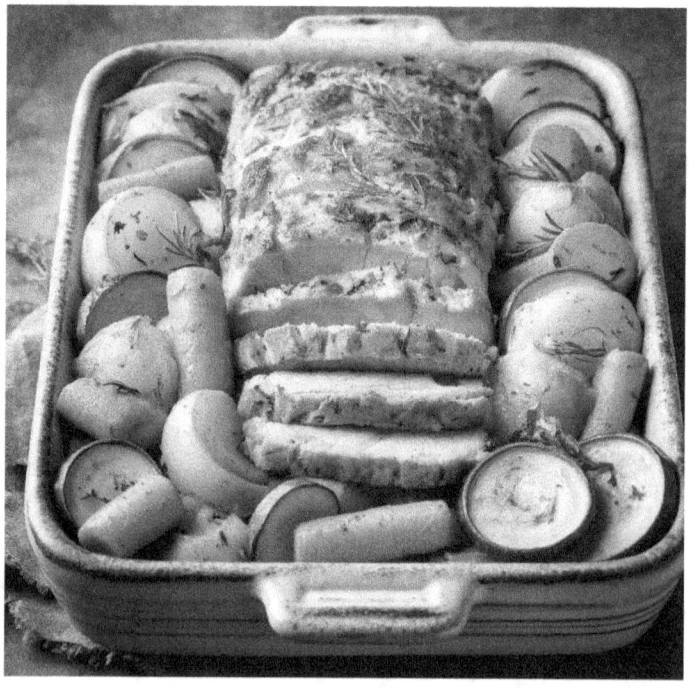

10. Pork and Mushroom Casserole

Ingredients
- 1 lb pork tenderloin, sliced
- 2 tablespoons olive oil
- 1 onion, chopped
- 2 cloves garlic, minced
- 8 oz mushrooms, sliced
- 1 cup low-sodium chicken broth
- 1/2 cup sour cream
- 1 teaspoon dried thyme

Instructions
1. Preheat the oven to 350°F (175°C).
2. Heat 1 tablespoon of olive oil in a large skillet over medium heat.
3. Add the sliced pork and cook until browned, about 5 minutes. Remove the pork and set aside.
4. Add the remaining olive oil to the skillet. Add the onion and garlic, and cook until soft, about 5 minutes.
5. Add the mushrooms and cook for another 5 minutes.
6. Stir in the chicken broth and bring to a boil.
7. Remove from heat and stir in the sour cream and thyme.
8. Return the pork to the skillet and mix well.
9. Transfer the mixture to a casserole dish and bake for 25-30 minutes, or until heated through.
10. Serve hot.

Nutrition Info per Serving
- Calories: 320
- Protein: 25g
- Fat: 20g
- Carbohydrates: 10g
- Fiber: 2g
- Sugars: 3g

Serves
4

Cooking Time
40 minutes

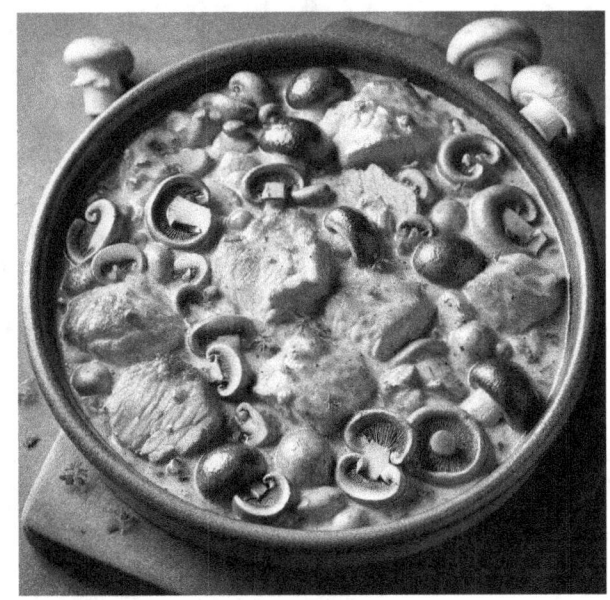

11. Pork and Carrot Salad

Ingredients
- 2 cups cooked pork tenderloin, sliced
- 2 large carrots, grated
- 1/4 cup raisins
- 1/4 cup sunflower seeds
- 1/2 cup plain Greek yogurt
- 1 tablespoon honey
- 1 teaspoon apple cider vinegar

Instructions
1. In a large bowl, combine the sliced pork, grated carrots, raisins, and sunflower seeds.
2. In a small bowl, mix the Greek yogurt, honey, and apple cider vinegar until well combined.
3. Pour the yogurt dressing over the salad and toss to coat.
4. Serve immediately or chill in the refrigerator until ready to serve.

Nutrition Info per Serving
- Calories: 250
- Protein: 20g
- Fat: 10g
- Carbohydrates: 20g
- Fiber: 4g
- Sugars: 15g

Serves
4

Cooking Time
10 minutes

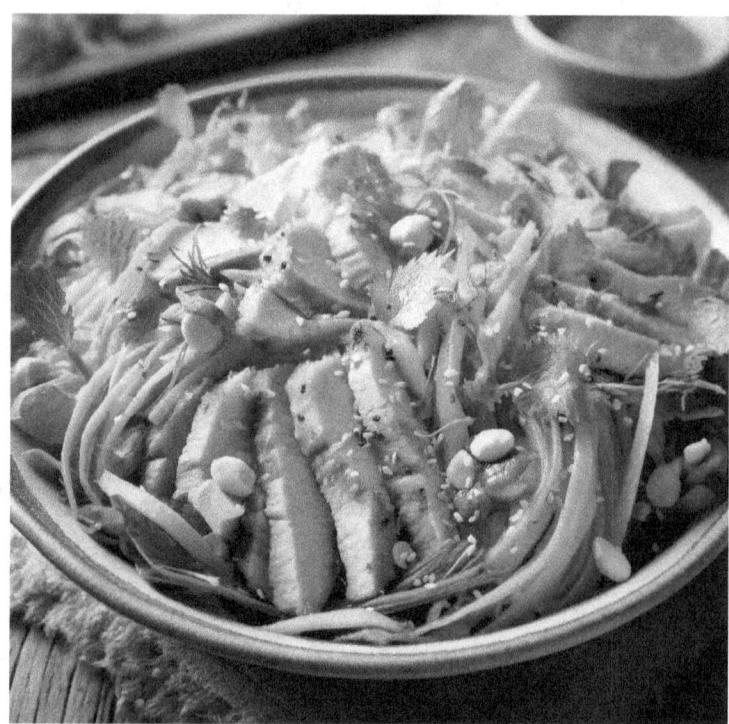

12. Pork and Vegetable Soup

Ingredients
- 1 tablespoon olive oil
- 1 onion, chopped
- 2 cloves garlic, minced
- 1 lb lean ground pork
- 4 cups low-sodium chicken broth
- 2 carrots, sliced
- 2 celery stalks, sliced
- 1 zucchini, diced
- 1 teaspoon dried thyme
- 1 teaspoon dried basil

Instructions
1. Heat the olive oil in a large pot over medium heat.
2. Add the onion and garlic, and cook until soft, about 5 minutes.
3. Add the ground pork and cook until browned, about 5-7 minutes.
4. Stir in the chicken broth, carrots, celery, zucchini, thyme, and basil.
5. Bring to a boil, then reduce heat and simmer for 20 minutes.
6. Serve hot.

Nutrition Info per Serving
- Calories: 280
- Protein: 20g
- Fat: 15g
- Carbohydrates: 15g
- Fiber: 4g
- Sugars: 5g

Serves
4

Cooking Time
30 minutes

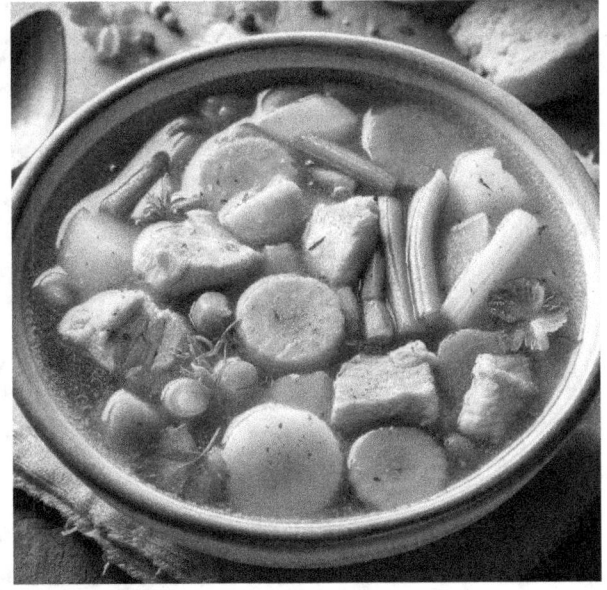

13. Pork and Spinach Soup

Ingredients
- 1 tablespoon olive oil
- 1 onion, chopped
- 2 cloves garlic, minced
- 1 lb lean ground pork
- 4 cups low-sodium chicken broth
- 2 cups fresh spinach, chopped
- 1 cup cooked brown rice
- 1 teaspoon ground cumin
- 1 teaspoon ground coriander

Instructions
1. Heat the olive oil in a large pot over medium heat.
2. Add the onion and garlic, and cook until soft, about 5 minutes.
3. Add the ground pork and cook until browned, about 5-7 minutes.
4. Stir in the chicken broth, spinach, cooked rice, cumin, and coriander.
5. Bring to a boil, then reduce heat and simmer for 10 minutes.
6. Serve hot.

Nutrition Info per Serving
- Calories: 300
- Protein: 20g
- Fat: 12g
- Carbohydrates: 25g
- Fiber: 4g
- Sugars: 3g

Serves
4

Cooking Time
25 minutes

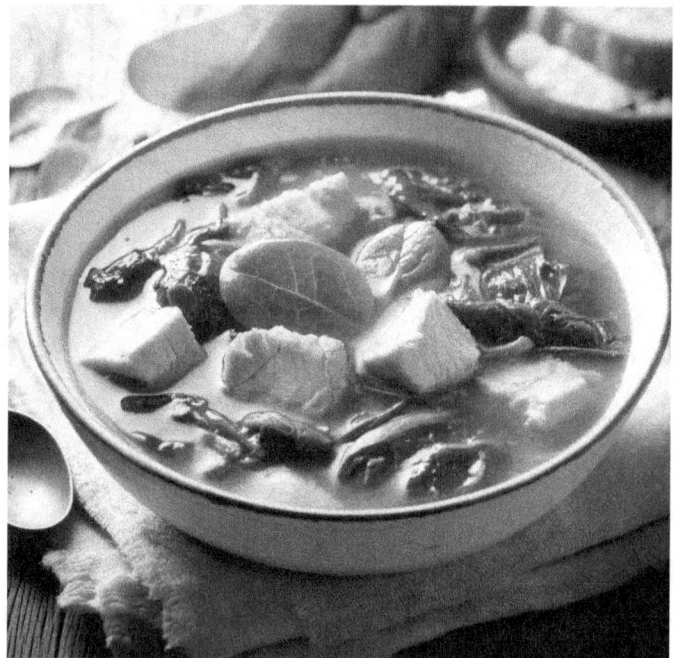

14. Pork and Soft Vegetable Casserole

Ingredients
- 1 lb pork tenderloin, sliced
- 2 tablespoons olive oil
- 1 onion, chopped
- 2 cloves garlic, minced
- 2 cups butternut squash, peeled and cubed
- 2 cups zucchini, sliced
- 1 cup low-sodium chicken broth
- 1/2 cup shredded mozzarella cheese
- 1 teaspoon dried thyme

Instructions
1. Preheat the oven to 350°F (175°C).
2. Heat 1 tablespoon of olive oil in a large skillet over medium heat.
3. Add the sliced pork and cook until browned, about 5 minutes. Remove the pork and set aside.
4. Add the remaining olive oil to the skillet. Add the onion and garlic, and cook until soft, about 5 minutes.
5. Add the butternut squash and zucchini, and cook for another 5 minutes.
6. Stir in the chicken broth and bring to a boil.
7. Remove from heat and stir in the shredded mozzarella cheese and thyme.
8. Return the pork to the skillet and mix well.
9. Transfer the mixture to a casserole dish and bake for 25-30 minutes, or until heated through.
10. Serve hot.

Nutrition Info per Serving
- Calories: 350
- Protein: 25g
- Fat: 20g
- Carbohydrates: 20g
- Fiber: 5g
- Sugars: 6g

Serves
4

Cooking Time
40 minutes

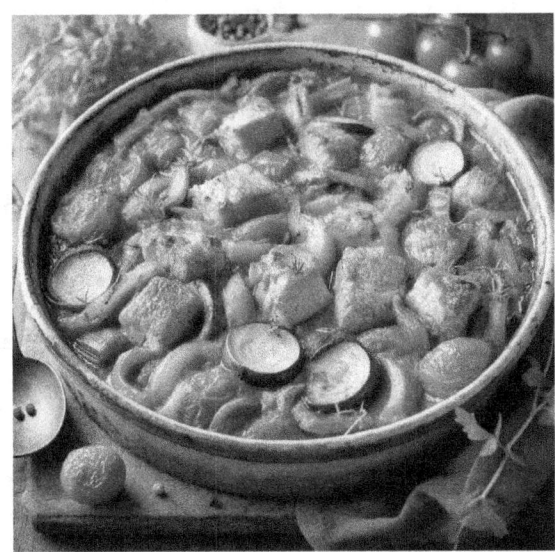

15. Beef and Apricot Salad

Ingredients

2 cups cooked beef sirloin, thinly sliced
1 cup dried apricots, chopped
1/2 cup red onion, thinly sliced
1/4 cup walnuts, chopped
1/4 cup fresh parsley, chopped
1/4 cup olive oil
2 tablespoons lemon juice
1 tablespoon honey
1 teaspoon ground cumin

Instructions

In a large bowl, combine the sliced beef, apricots, red onion, walnuts, and parsley.
In a small bowl, whisk together the olive oil, lemon juice, honey, and ground cumin.
Pour the dressing over the salad and toss to coat.
Serve immediately or chill in the refrigerator until ready to serve.

Nutrition Info per Serving

Calories: 350
Protein: 25g
Fat: 20g
Carbohydrates: 25g
Fiber: 4g
Sugars: 15g
Serves
4

Cooking Time

10 minutes

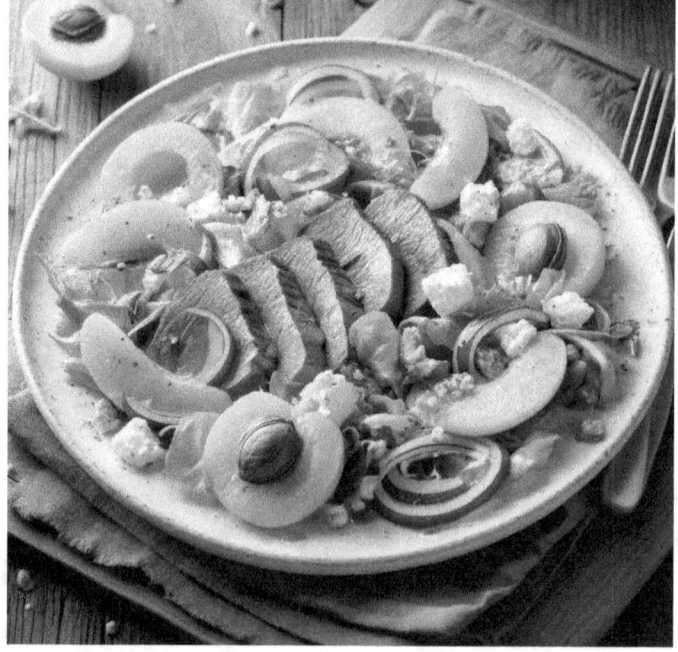

16. Beef and Vegetable Bake

Ingredients
- 1 lb beef sirloin, cut into cubes
- 2 tablespoons olive oil
- 2 cups broccoli florets
- 2 cups cauliflower florets
- 1 red bell pepper, sliced
- 1 teaspoon dried oregano
- 1 teaspoon dried basil

Instructions
1. Preheat the oven to 375°F (190°C).
2. Place the beef cubes in a baking dish and brush with 1 tablespoon of olive oil.
3. In a large bowl, toss the broccoli, cauliflower, and red bell pepper with the remaining olive oil, oregano, and basil.
4. Arrange the vegetables around the beef in the baking dish.
5. Bake for 25-30 minutes, or until the beef is cooked through and the vegetables are tender.
6. Let it rest for 5 minutes before serving.

Nutrition Info per Serving
- Calories: 300
- Protein: 25g
- Fat: 15g
- Carbohydrates: 15g
- Fiber: 5g
- Sugars: 5g

Serves
4

Cooking Time
35 minutes

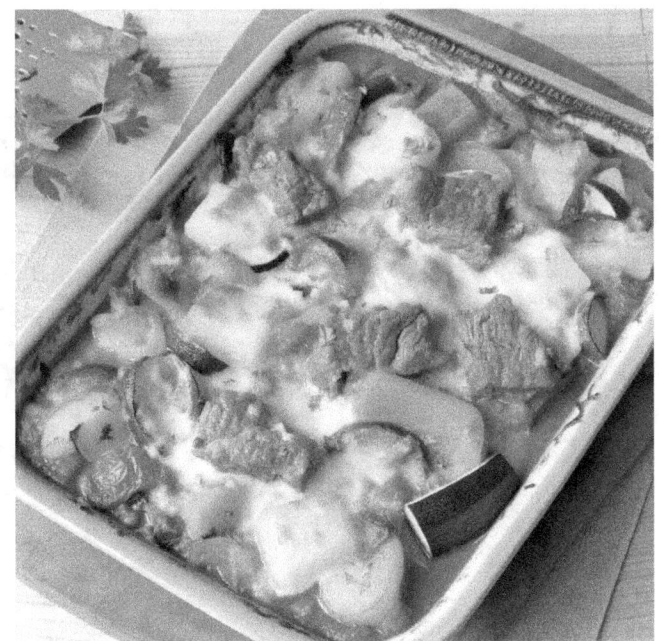

17. Beef and Pumpkin Mash

Ingredients
- 1 lb beef sirloin, sliced
- 2 tablespoons olive oil
- 2 cups pumpkin, peeled and cubed
- 1/4 cup milk (dairy or plant-based)
- 1 tablespoon butter
- 1 teaspoon ground nutmeg

Instructions
1. Preheat the oven to 375°F (190°C).
2. Place the sliced beef on a baking sheet and brush with 1 tablespoon of olive oil. Bake for 20-25 minutes, or until the beef is cooked through.
3. While the beef is baking, steam the pumpkin cubes until tender, about 10-15 minutes.
4. In a blender or food processor, combine the steamed pumpkin, milk, butter, and ground nutmeg. Blend until smooth.
5. Serve the baked beef with a side of pumpkin mash.

Nutrition Info per Serving
- Calories: 350
- Protein: 25g
- Fat: 18g
- Carbohydrates: 20g
- Fiber: 4g
- Sugars: 6g

Serves
4

Cooking Time
30 minutes

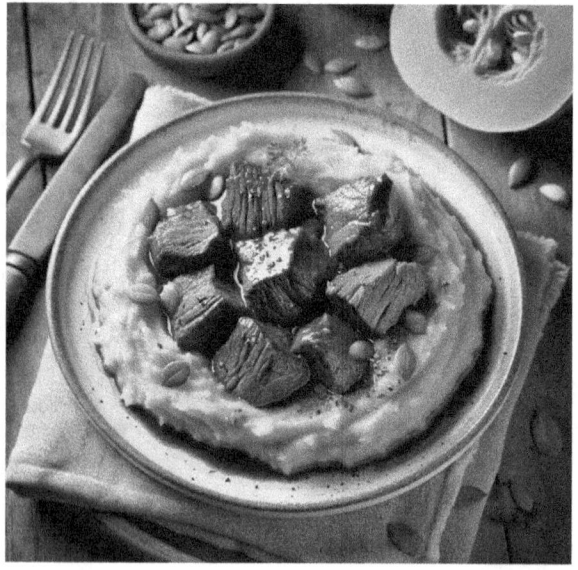

18. Beef and Mashed Potatoes

Ingredients
- 1 lb beef sirloin, sliced
- 2 tablespoons olive oil
- 4 large potatoes, peeled and cubed
- 1/2 cup milk (dairy or plant-based)
- 1/4 cup butter
- 1 teaspoon garlic powder

Instructions
1. Preheat the oven to 375°F (190°C).
2. Place the sliced beef on a baking sheet and brush with 1 tablespoon of olive oil. Bake for 20-25 minutes, or until the beef is cooked through.
3. While the beef is baking, boil the potatoes in a large pot of water until tender, about 15 minutes.
4. Drain the potatoes and return them to the pot.
5. Add the milk, butter, and garlic powder to the potatoes. Mash until smooth.
6. Serve the baked beef with a side of mashed potatoes.

Nutrition Info per Serving
- Calories: 400
- Protein: 25g
- Fat: 20g
- Carbohydrates: 30g
- Fiber: 4g
- Sugars: 3g

Serves
4

Cooking Time
30 minutes

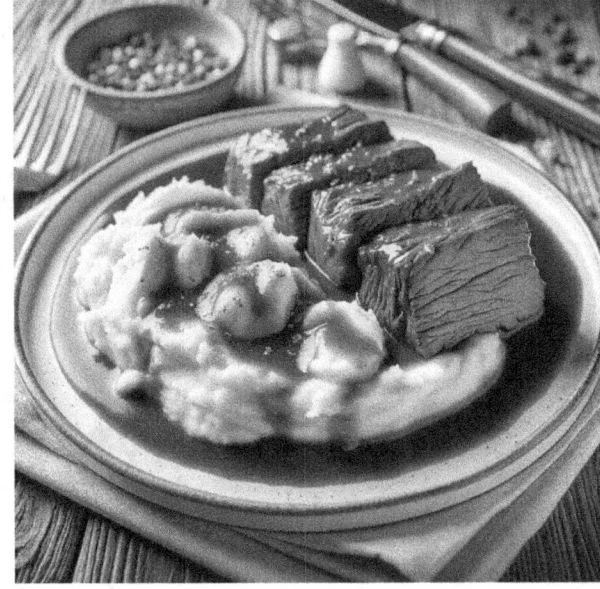

19. Beef and Carrot Puree

Ingredients
- 1 lb beef sirloin, sliced
- 2 tablespoons olive oil
- 4 large carrots, peeled and chopped
- 1/4 cup plain Greek yogurt
- 1 teaspoon ground cumin

Instructions
1. Preheat the oven to 375°F (190°C).
2. Place the sliced beef on a baking sheet and brush with 1 tablespoon of olive oil. Bake for 20-25 minutes, or until the beef is cooked through.
3. While the beef is baking, steam the carrots until tender, about 10-15 minutes.
4. In a blender or food processor, combine the steamed carrots, Greek yogurt, and ground cumin. Blend until smooth.
5. Serve the baked beef with a side of carrot puree.

Nutrition Info per Serving
- Calories: 300
- Protein: 25g
- Fat: 15g
- Carbohydrates: 15g
- Fiber: 4g
- Sugars: 7g

Serves
4

Cooking Time
30 minutes

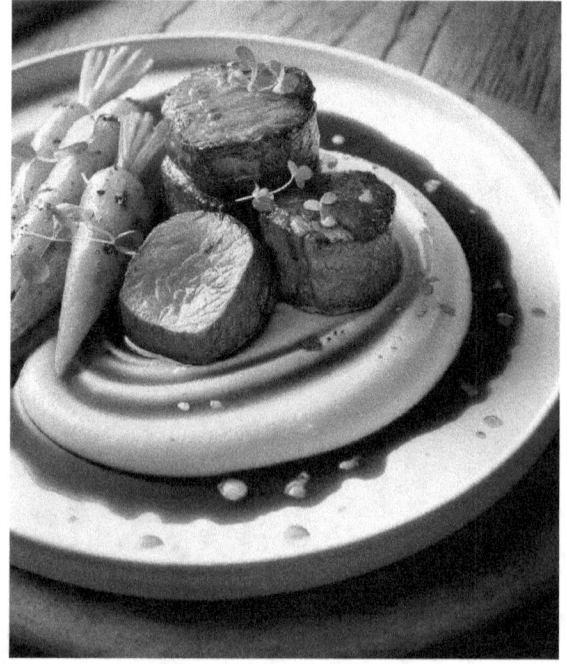

Fish and Seafood Recipes

1. Baked Salmon
Ingredients
- 4 salmon fillets
- 2 tablespoons olive oil
- 2 tablespoons lemon juice
- 1 tablespoon dried dill
- 1 teaspoon garlic powder
- 1 lemon, sliced

Instructions
1. Preheat the oven to 375°F (190°C).
2. In a small bowl, mix olive oil, lemon juice, dried dill, and garlic powder.
3. Place the salmon fillets on a baking sheet and brush with the olive oil mixture.
4. Arrange lemon slices on top of the salmon.
5. Bake for 20-25 minutes, or until the salmon is cooked through.
6. Serve immediately.

Nutrition Info per Serving
- Calories: 300
- Protein: 25g
- Fat: 20g
- Carbohydrates: 2g
- Fiber: 0g
- Sugars: 0g

Serves
4

Cooking Time
25 minutes

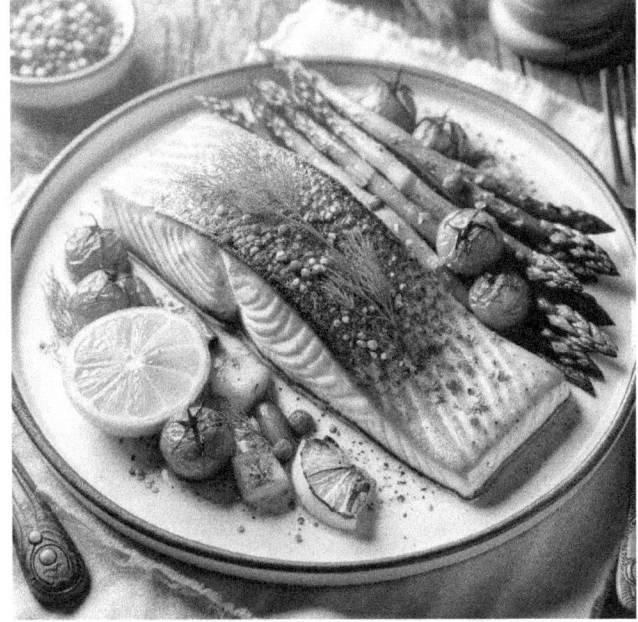

2. Grilled Cod

Ingredients
- 4 cod fillets
- 2 tablespoons olive oil
- 1 tablespoon lemon juice
- 1 teaspoon dried thyme
- 1 teaspoon garlic powder

Instructions
1. Preheat the grill to medium-high heat.
2. In a small bowl, mix olive oil, lemon juice, dried thyme, and garlic powder.
3. Brush the cod fillets with the olive oil mixture.
4. Grill the cod fillets for 4-5 minutes per side, or until the fish is opaque and flakes easily with a fork.
5. Serve immediately.

Nutrition Info per Serving
- Calories: 180
- Protein: 25g
- Fat: 8g
- Carbohydrates: 1g
- Fiber: 0g
- Sugars: 0g

Serves
4

Cooking Time
10 minutes

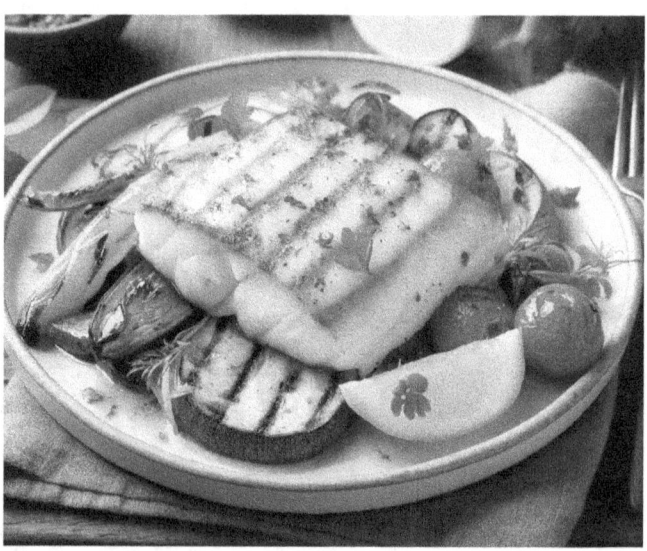

3. Baked Tilapia

Ingredients
- 4 tilapia fillets
- 2 tablespoons olive oil
- 1 teaspoon paprika
- 1 teaspoon garlic powder
- 1 teaspoon dried parsley

Instructions
1. Preheat the oven to 375°F (190°C).
2. Place the tilapia fillets on a baking sheet and brush with olive oil.
3. In a small bowl, mix paprika, garlic powder, and dried parsley.
4. Sprinkle the spice mixture evenly over the tilapia fillets.
5. Bake for 15-20 minutes, or until the fish is opaque and flakes easily with a fork.
6. Serve immediately.

Nutrition Info per Serving
- Calories: 200
- Protein: 22g
- Fat: 10g
- Carbohydrates: 1g
- Fiber: 0g
- Sugars: 0g

Serves
4

Cooking Time
20 minutes

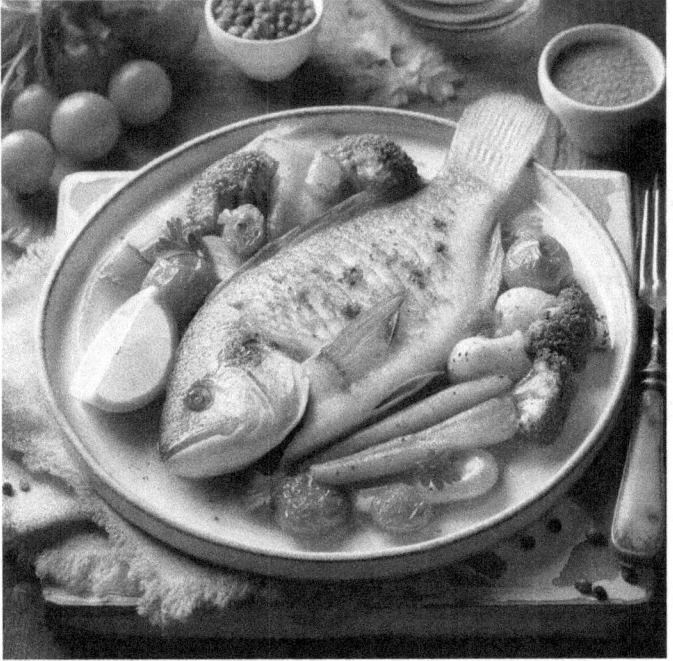

4. Salmon Cakes

Ingredients
- 1 lb cooked salmon, flaked
- 1/2 cup breadcrumbs
- 1/4 cup mayonnaise
- 1 egg
- 2 tablespoons green onions, finely chopped
- 1 tablespoon lemon juice
- 1 teaspoon dried dill
- 2 tablespoons olive oil for frying

Instructions
1. In a large bowl, combine the flaked salmon, breadcrumbs, mayonnaise, egg, green onions, lemon juice, and dried dill.
2. Form the mixture into patties.
3. Heat the olive oil in a large skillet over medium heat.
4. Cook the salmon cakes for 3-4 minutes per side, or until golden brown and heated through.
5. Serve immediately.

Nutrition Info per Serving
- Calories: 250
- Protein: 20g
- Fat: 15g
- Carbohydrates: 10g
- Fiber: 1g
- Sugars: 1g

Serves
4

Cooking Time
15 minutes

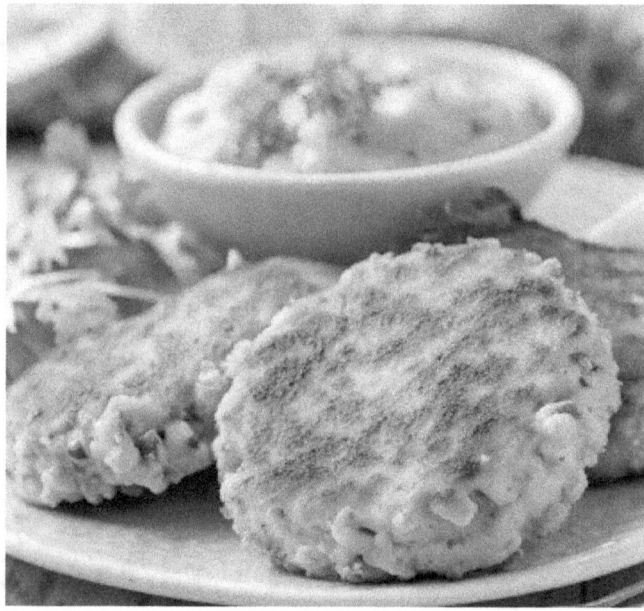

5. Fish Tacos

Ingredients
- 1 lb white fish fillets (such as cod or tilapia), cut into strips
- 2 tablespoons olive oil
- 1 teaspoon ground cumin
- 1 teaspoon paprika
- 8 small corn tortillas
- 1 cup shredded lettuce
- 1/2 cup diced tomatoes
- 1/4 cup plain Greek yogurt
- 1 tablespoon lime juice

Instructions
1. Preheat the oven to 375°F (190°C).
2. In a small bowl, mix olive oil, ground cumin, and paprika.
3. Brush the fish strips with the olive oil mixture.
4. Place the fish strips on a baking sheet and bake for 10-12 minutes, or until the fish is opaque and flakes easily with a fork.
5. Warm the tortillas in a skillet over medium heat.
6. Fill each tortilla with the baked fish, shredded lettuce, and diced tomatoes.
7. In a small bowl, mix Greek yogurt and lime juice.
8. Drizzle the yogurt sauce over the tacos.
9. Serve immediately.

Nutrition Info per Serving
- Calories: 200
- Protein: 20g
- Fat: 10g
- Carbohydrates: 15g
- Fiber: 2g
- Sugars: 2g

Serves
4

Cooking Time
15 minutes

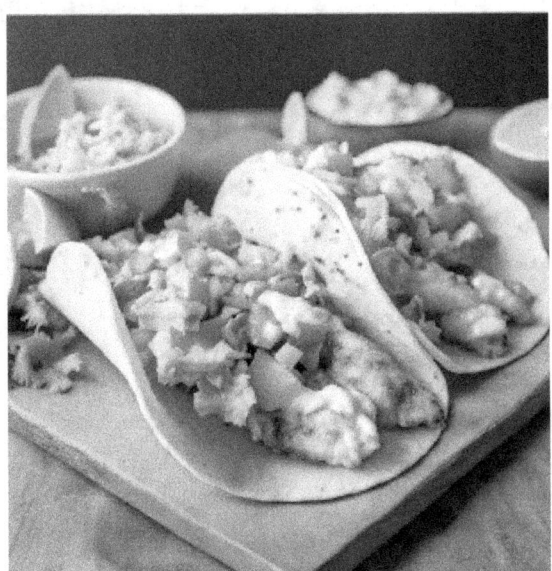

6. Cod and Sweet Potato Bake

Ingredients
- 4 cod fillets
- 2 large sweet potatoes, peeled and cubed
- 2 tablespoons olive oil
- 1 teaspoon ground paprika
- 1 teaspoon garlic powder
- 1 teaspoon dried thyme

Instructions
1. Preheat the oven to 375°F (190°C).
2. In a large bowl, toss the sweet potato cubes with olive oil, paprika, garlic powder, and dried thyme.
3. Place the cod fillets and seasoned sweet potatoes in a baking dish.
4. Bake for 25-30 minutes, or until the fish is opaque and flakes easily with a fork, and the sweet potatoes are tender.
5. Serve immediately.

Nutrition Info per Serving
- Calories: 280
- Protein: 25g
- Fat: 10g
- Carbohydrates: 25g
- Fiber: 4g
- Sugars: 6g

Serves
4

Cooking Time
30 minutes

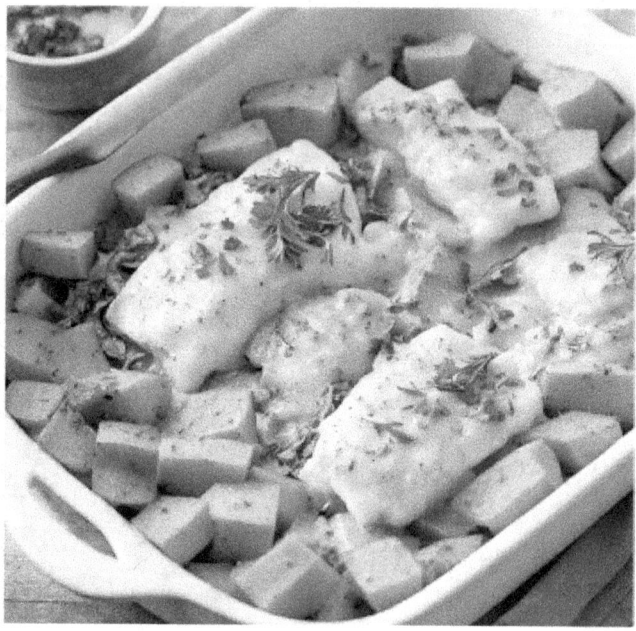

7. Salmon and Spinach Frittata

Ingredients
- 6 large eggs
- 1/2 cup milk (dairy or plant-based)
- 1 cup cooked salmon, flaked
- 1 cup fresh spinach, chopped
- 1/2 cup shredded mozzarella cheese
- 1 teaspoon dried dill

Instructions
1. Preheat the oven to 375°F (190°C). Grease a baking dish.
2. In a large bowl, whisk together eggs and milk.
3. Stir in flaked salmon, spinach, mozzarella cheese, and dried dill.
4. Pour the mixture into the prepared baking dish.
5. Bake for 25-30 minutes, or until the frittata is set and golden brown.
6. Let it cool for a few minutes before slicing and serving.

Nutrition Info per Serving
- Calories: 250
- Protein: 20g
- Fat: 15g
- Carbohydrates: 3g
- Fiber: 1g
- Sugars: 1g

Serves
4

Cooking Time
35 minutes

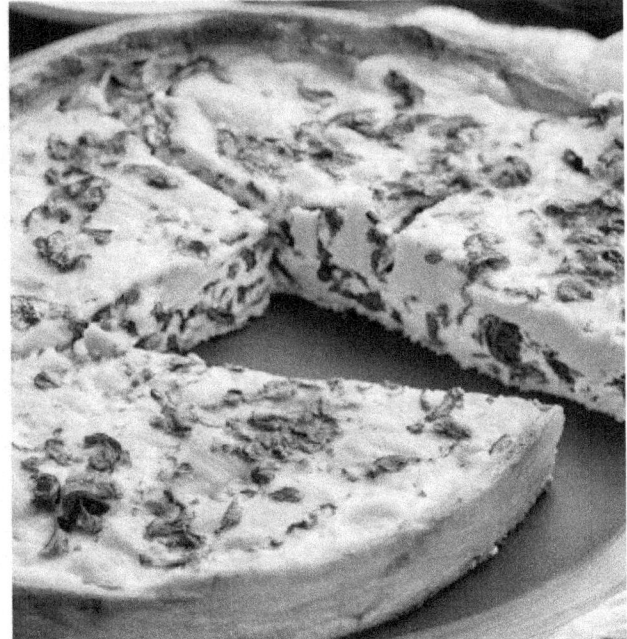

8. Grilled Halibut

Ingredients
- 4 halibut fillets
- 2 tablespoons olive oil
- 1 tablespoon lemon juice
- 1 teaspoon dried basil
- 1 teaspoon garlic powder

Instructions
1. Preheat the grill to medium-high heat.
2. In a small bowl, mix olive oil, lemon juice, dried basil, and garlic powder.
3. Brush the halibut fillets with the olive oil mixture.
4. Grill the halibut fillets for 4-5 minutes per side, or until the fish is opaque and flakes easily with a fork.
5. Serve immediately.

Nutrition Info per Serving
- Calories: 220
- Protein: 25g
- Fat: 12g
- Carbohydrates: 1g
- Fiber: 0g
- Sugars: 0g

Serves
4

Cooking Time
10 minutes

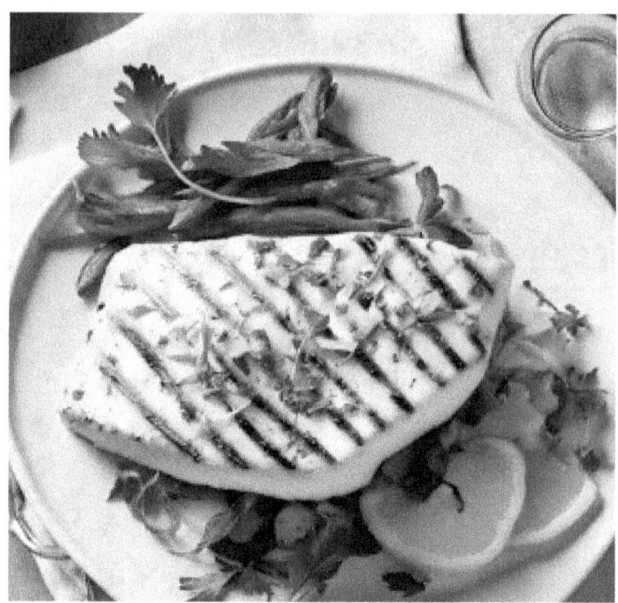

9. Cod and Bell Pepper Stir-Fry

Ingredients
- 4 cod fillets, cut into chunks
- 2 tablespoons olive oil
- 1 red bell pepper, sliced
- 1 yellow bell pepper, sliced
- 2 cloves garlic, minced
- 1 teaspoon ground ginger
- 1 tablespoon low-sodium soy sauce

Instructions
1. Heat 1 tablespoon of olive oil in a large skillet over medium heat.
2. Add the cod chunks and cook until opaque and flakes easily with a fork, about 5-7 minutes. Remove the cod and set aside.
3. Add the remaining olive oil to the skillet. Add the bell peppers and garlic, and cook until soft, about 5 minutes.
4. Stir in the ground ginger and soy sauce.
5. Return the cod to the skillet and cook for another 2-3 minutes, until everything is heated through.
6. Serve immediately.

Nutrition Info per Serving
- Calories: 200
- Protein: 22g
- Fat: 10g
- Carbohydrates: 5g
- Fiber: 2g
- Sugars: 2g

Serves
4

Cooking Time
15 minutes

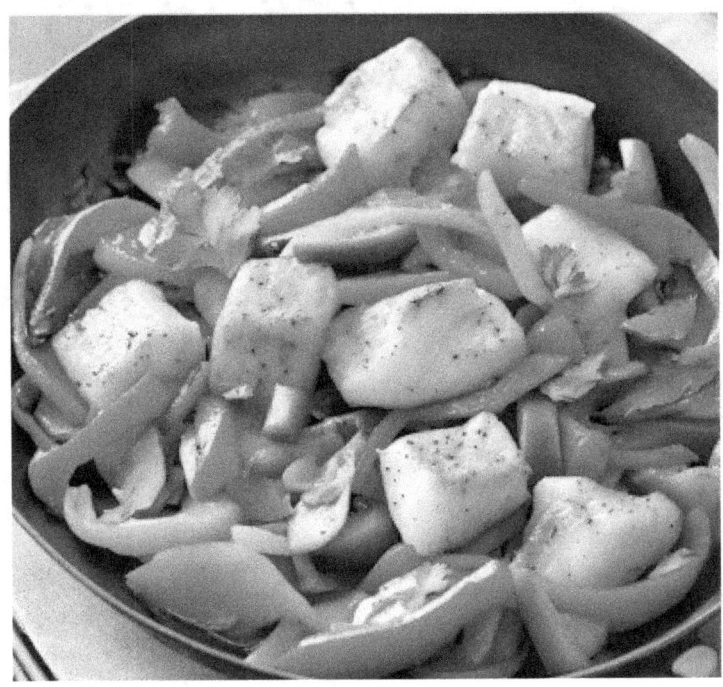

10. Salmon and Butternut Squash Stew

Ingredients

- 1 lb salmon fillets, cut into chunks
- 2 tablespoons olive oil
- 1 onion, chopped
- 2 cloves garlic, minced
- 4 cups low-sodium vegetable broth
- 2 cups butternut squash, peeled and cubed
- 1 teaspoon dried thyme
- 1 teaspoon ground cumin

Instructions

1. Heat 1 tablespoon of olive oil in a large pot over medium heat.
2. Add the onion and garlic, and cook until soft, about 5 minutes.
3. Add the vegetable broth, butternut squash, thyme, and cumin. Bring to a boil, then reduce heat and simmer for 20 minutes.
4. While the stew is simmering, heat the remaining olive oil in a skillet over medium heat. Add the salmon chunks and cook until opaque and flakes easily with a fork, about 5-7 minutes.
5. Add the cooked salmon to the stew and simmer for another 5 minutes.
6. Serve hot.

Nutrition Info per Serving

- Calories: 300
- Protein: 25g
- Fat: 15g
- Carbohydrates: 15g
- Fiber: 3g
- Sugars: 5g

Serves

4

Cooking Time

35 minutes

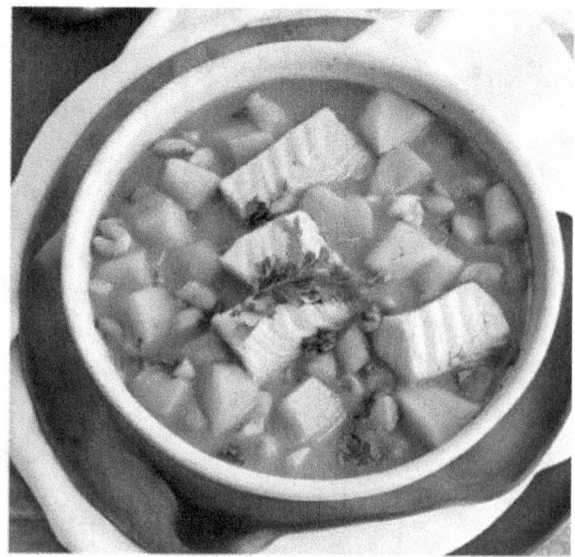

11. Grilled Sole

Ingredients
- 4 sole fillets
- 2 tablespoons olive oil
- 1 tablespoon lemon juice
- 1 teaspoon dried thyme
- 1 teaspoon garlic powder

Instructions
1. Preheat the grill to medium-high heat.
2. In a small bowl, mix olive oil, lemon juice, dried thyme, and garlic powder.
3. Brush the sole fillets with the olive oil mixture.
4. Grill the sole fillets for 3-4 minutes per side, or until the fish is opaque and flakes easily with a fork.
5. Serve immediately.

Nutrition Info per Serving
- Calories: 180
- Protein: 22g
- Fat: 10g
- Carbohydrates: 1g
- Fiber: 0g
- Sugars: 0g

Serves
4

Cooking Time
10 minutes

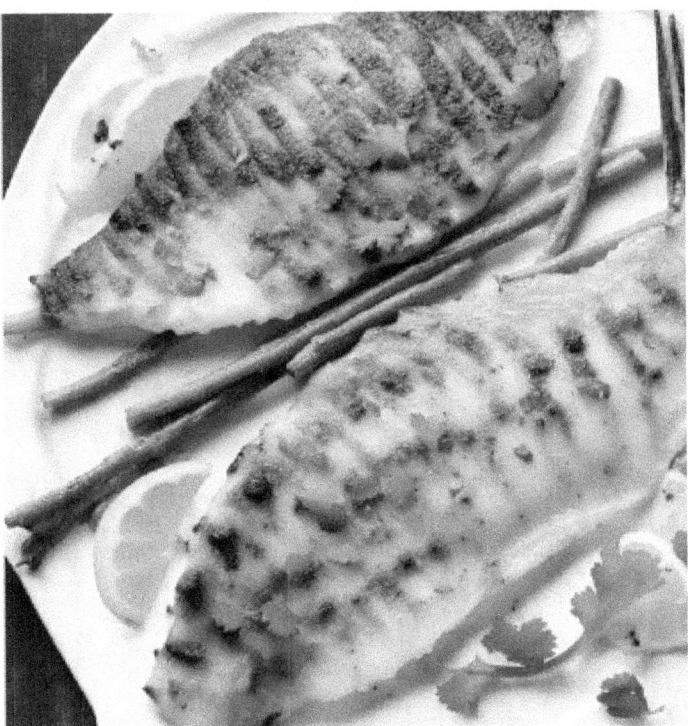

12. Grilled Mahi Mahi

Ingredients
- 4 mahi mahi fillets
- 2 tablespoons olive oil
- 1 tablespoon lime juice
- 1 teaspoon ground cumin
- 1 teaspoon paprika

Instructions
1. Preheat the grill to medium-high heat.
2. In a small bowl, mix olive oil, lime juice, ground cumin, and paprika.
3. Brush the mahi mahi fillets with the olive oil mixture.
4. Grill the mahi mahi fillets for 4-5 minutes per side, or until the fish is opaque and flakes easily with a fork.
5. Serve immediately.

Nutrition Info per Serving
- Calories: 200
- Protein: 25g
- Fat: 10g
- Carbohydrates: 1g
- Fiber: 0g
- Sugars: 0g

Serves
4

Cooking Time
10 minutes

13. Baked Flounder

Ingredients
- 4 flounder fillets
- 2 tablespoons olive oil
- 1 teaspoon paprika
- 1 teaspoon garlic powder
- 1 teaspoon dried parsley

Instructions
1. Preheat the oven to 375°F (190°C).
2. Place the flounder fillets on a baking sheet and brush with olive oil.
3. In a small bowl, mix paprika, garlic powder, and dried parsley.
4. Sprinkle the spice mixture evenly over the flounder fillets.
5. Bake for 15-20 minutes, or until the fish is opaque and flakes easily with a fork.
6. Serve immediately.

Nutrition Info per Serving
- Calories: 200
- Protein: 22g
- Fat: 10g
- Carbohydrates: 1g
- Fiber: 0g
- Sugars: 0g

Serves
4

Cooking Time
20 minutes

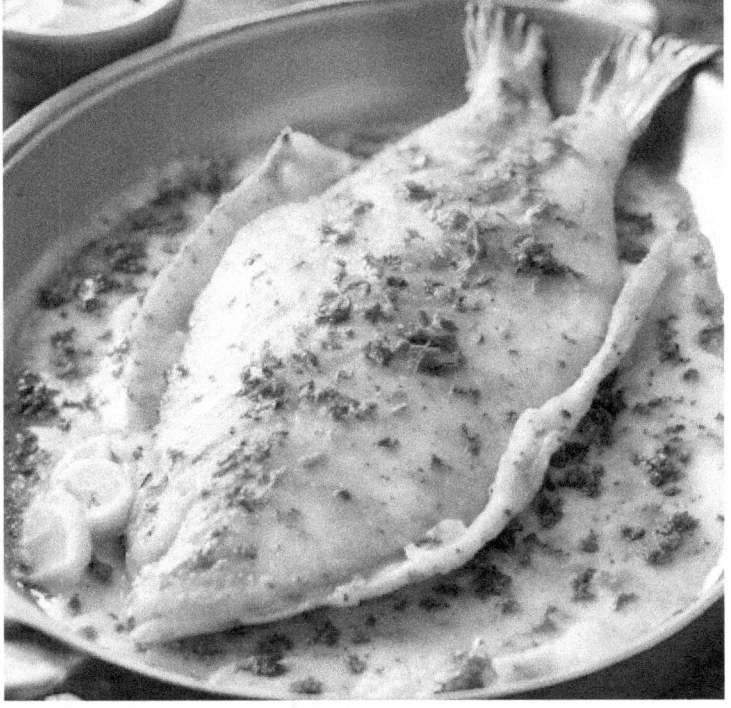

14. Shrimp and Rice Soup

Ingredients
- 1 tablespoon olive oil
- 1 onion, chopped
- 2 cloves garlic, minced
- 1 lb shrimp, peeled and deveined
- 4 cups low-sodium chicken broth
- 1 cup cooked brown rice
- 1 carrot, sliced
- 1 celery stalk, sliced
- 1 teaspoon dried thyme

Instructions
1. Heat the olive oil in a large pot over medium heat.
2. Add the onion and garlic, and cook until soft, about 5 minutes.
3. Add the chicken broth, cooked rice, carrot, celery, and thyme. Bring to a boil, then reduce heat and simmer for 10 minutes.
4. Add the shrimp and cook for another 5 minutes, or until the shrimp are pink and cooked through.
5. Serve hot.

Nutrition Info per Serving
- Calories: 250
- Protein: 20g
- Fat: 8g
- Carbohydrates: 25g
- Fiber: 2g
- Sugars: 3g

Serves
4

Cooking Time
20 minutes

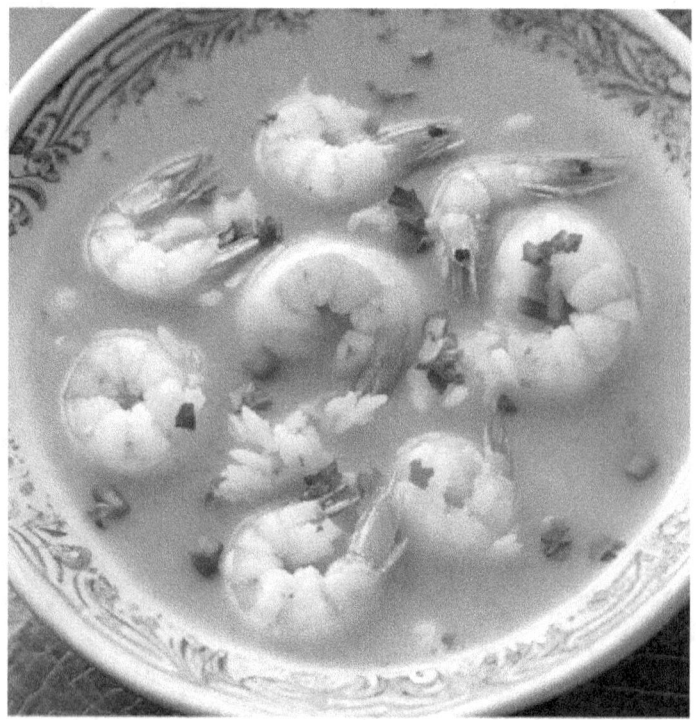

15. Grilled Shrimp Skewers

Ingredients
- 1 lb shrimp, peeled and deveined
- 2 tablespoons olive oil
- 1 tablespoon lemon juice
- 1 teaspoon dried oregano
- 1 teaspoon garlic powder

Instructions
1. Preheat the grill to medium-high heat.
2. In a small bowl, mix olive oil, lemon juice, dried oregano, and garlic powder.
3. Thread the shrimp onto skewers and brush with the olive oil mixture.
4. Grill the shrimp skewers for 2-3 minutes per side, or until the shrimp are pink and cooked through.
5. Serve immediately.

Nutrition Info per Serving
- Calories: 180
- Protein: 20g
- Fat: 10g
- Carbohydrates: 1g
- Fiber: 0g
- Sugars: 0g

Serves
4

Cooking Time
10 minutes

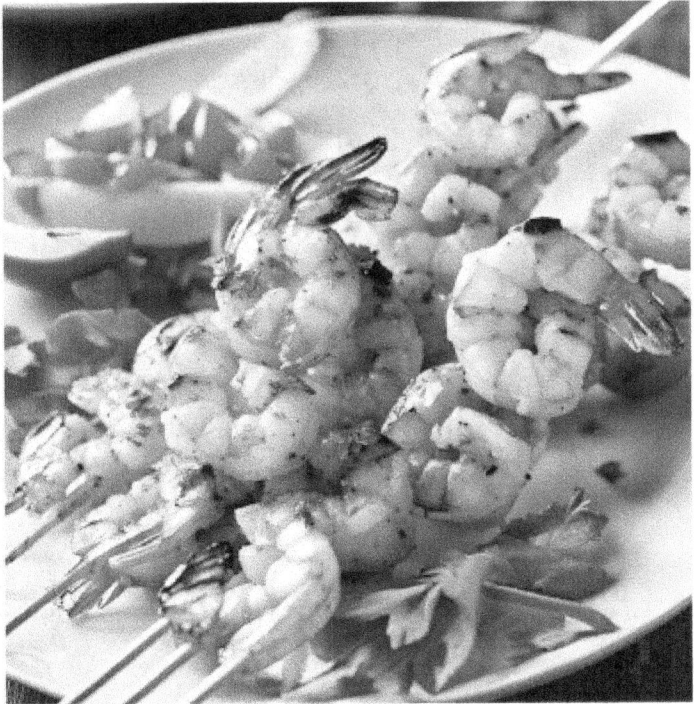

16. Baked Scallops

Ingredients
- 1 lb scallops
- 2 tablespoons olive oil
- 1 teaspoon garlic powder
- 1 teaspoon dried parsley
- 1/4 cup grated Parmesan cheese

Instructions
1. Preheat the oven to 400°F (200°C).
2. Place the scallops in a baking dish and drizzle with olive oil.
3. In a small bowl, mix garlic powder, dried parsley, and Parmesan cheese.
4. Sprinkle the spice mixture evenly over the scallops.
5. Bake for 12-15 minutes, or until the scallops are opaque and cooked through.
6. Serve immediately.

Nutrition Info per Serving
- Calories: 220
- Protein: 25g
- Fat: 12g
- Carbohydrates: 2g
- Fiber: 0g
- Sugars: 0g

Serves
4

Cooking Time
15 minutes

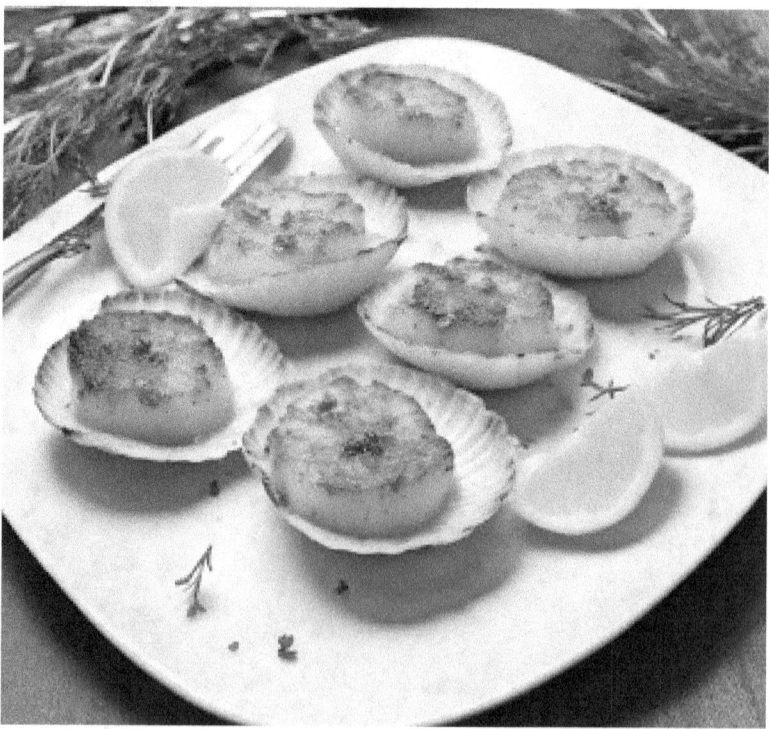

17. Shrimp and Rice Casserole

Ingredients
- 1 lb shrimp, peeled and deveined
- 1 cup cooked brown rice
- 1 cup broccoli florets
- 1 cup shredded cheddar cheese
- 1/2 cup plain Greek yogurt
- 1 teaspoon garlic powder

Instructions
1. Preheat the oven to 375°F (190°C).
2. In a large bowl, combine shrimp, cooked rice, broccoli florets, cheddar cheese, Greek yogurt, and garlic powder.
3. Transfer the mixture to a greased casserole dish.
4. Bake for 20-25 minutes, or until the shrimp are pink and cooked through, and the casserole is heated through.
5. Serve hot.

Nutrition Info per Serving
- Calories: 300
- Protein: 25g
- Fat: 12g
- Carbohydrates: 25g
- Fiber: 3g
- Sugars: 2g

Serves
4

Cooking Time
25 minutes

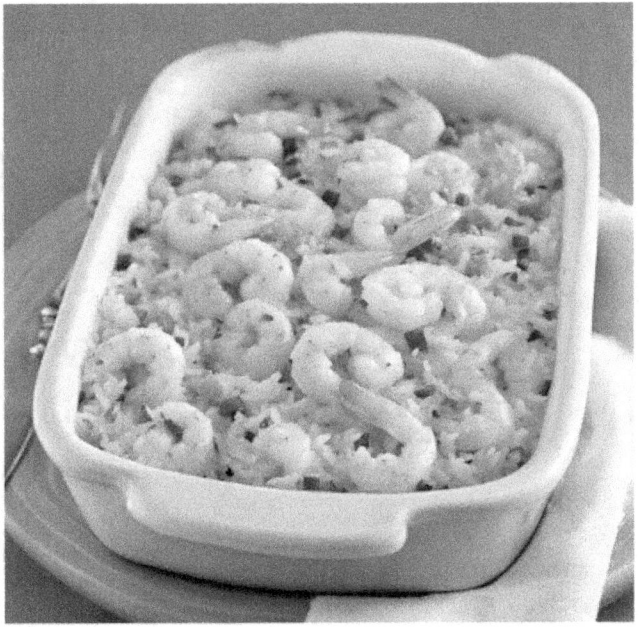

18. Grilled Scallops with Rice

Ingredients
- 1 lb scallops
- 2 tablespoons olive oil
- 1 teaspoon lemon juice
- 1 teaspoon dried thyme
- 1 cup cooked brown rice

Instructions
1. Preheat the grill to medium-high heat.
2. In a small bowl, mix olive oil, lemon juice, and dried thyme.
3. Brush the scallops with the olive oil mixture.
4. Grill the scallops for 2-3 minutes per side, or until the scallops are opaque and cooked through.
5. Serve the grilled scallops with a side of cooked brown rice.

Nutrition Info per Serving
- Calories: 300
- Protein: 25g
- Fat: 12g
- Carbohydrates: 25g
- Fiber: 2g
- Sugars: 1g

Serves
4

Cooking Time
10 minutes

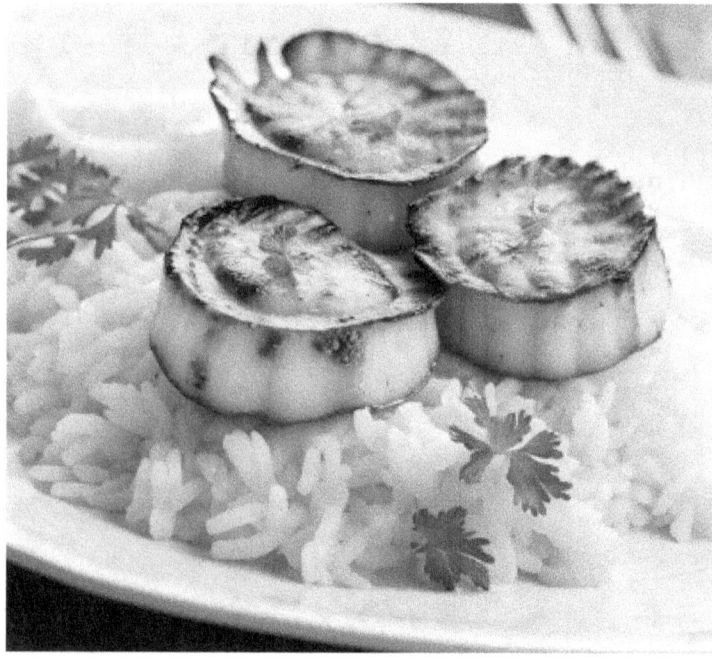

19. Grilled Shrimp with Bell Peppers

Ingredients
- 1 lb shrimp, peeled and deveined
- 2 bell peppers (any color), sliced
- 2 tablespoons olive oil
- 1 teaspoon ground cumin
- 1 teaspoon garlic powder

Instructions
1. Preheat the grill to medium-high heat.
2. In a large bowl, toss the shrimp and bell peppers with olive oil, ground cumin, and garlic powder.
3. Thread the shrimp and bell peppers onto skewers.
4. Grill the skewers for 2-3 minutes per side, or until the shrimp are pink and cooked through, and the bell peppers are tender.
5. Serve immediately.

Nutrition Info per Serving
- Calories: 200
- Protein: 20g
- Fat: 10g
- Carbohydrates: 6g
- Fiber: 2g
- Sugars: 3g

Serves
4

Cooking Time
15 minutes

20. Shrimp and Zucchini Soup

Ingredients
- 1 tablespoon olive oil
- 1 onion, chopped
- 2 cloves garlic, minced
- 1 lb shrimp, peeled and deveined
- 4 cups low-sodium chicken broth
- 2 zucchinis, diced
- 1 teaspoon dried basil

Instructions
1. Heat the olive oil in a large pot over medium heat.
2. Add the onion and garlic, and cook until soft, about 5 minutes.
3. Add the chicken broth and bring to a boil.
4. Add the shrimp, zucchini, and basil. Reduce heat and simmer for 10 minutes, or until the shrimp are pink and cooked through.
5. Serve hot.

Nutrition Info per Serving
- Calories: 200
- Protein: 20g
- Fat: 8g
- Carbohydrates: 8g
- Fiber: 2g
- Sugars: 4g

Serves
4

Cooking Time
20 minutes

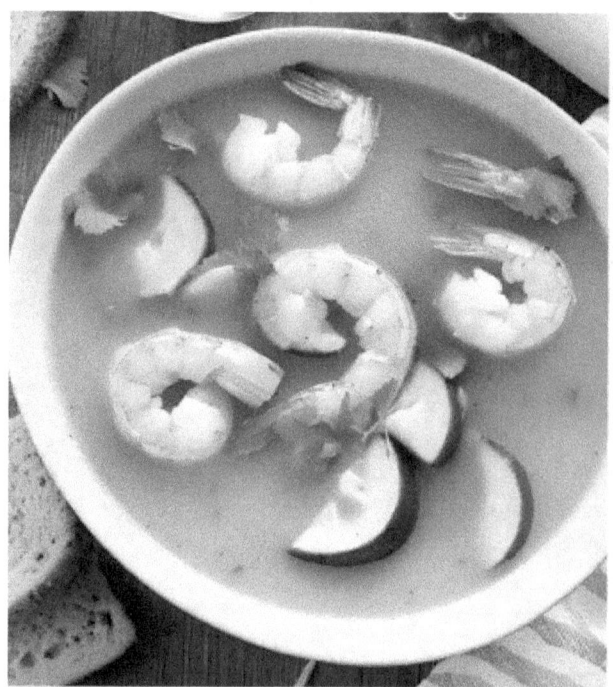

Snacks & Sides Recipes

1. Yogurt with Honey
Ingredients
- 2 cups plain Greek yogurt
- 2 tablespoons honey

Instructions
1. Divide the Greek yogurt into two serving bowls.
2. Drizzle 1 tablespoon of honey over each bowl of yogurt.
3. Serve immediately.

Nutrition Info per Serving
- Calories: 150
- Protein: 15g
- Fat: 4g
- Carbohydrates: 15g
- Fiber: 0g
- Sugars: 15g

Serves
2

Cooking Time
5 minutes

2. Rice Cakes with Avocado

Ingredients
- 4 plain rice cakes
- 2 ripe avocados
- 1 tablespoon lemon juice
- 1 teaspoon garlic powder

Instructions
1. In a bowl, mash the avocados with lemon juice and garlic powder until smooth.
2. Spread the avocado mixture evenly on each rice cake.
3. Serve immediately.

Nutrition Info per Serving
- Calories: 180
- Protein: 2g
- Fat: 15g
- Carbohydrates: 12g
- Fiber: 7g
- Sugars: 0g

Serves
4

Cooking Time
5 minutes

3. Oatmeal Cookies

Ingredients
- 1 cup rolled oats
- 1/2 cup whole wheat flour
- 1/2 teaspoon baking powder
- 1/2 teaspoon ground cinnamon
- 1/4 cup honey
- 1/4 cup unsweetened applesauce
- 1 large egg
- 1 teaspoon vanilla extract

Instructions
1. Preheat the oven to 350°F (175°C). Line a baking sheet with parchment paper.
2. In a large bowl, combine the oats, whole wheat flour, baking powder, and cinnamon.
3. In another bowl, mix the honey, applesauce, egg, and vanilla extract until well combined.
4. Pour the wet ingredients into the dry ingredients and stir until just combined.
5. Drop spoonfuls of the dough onto the prepared baking sheet.
6. Bake for 10-12 minutes, or until the edges are golden brown.
7. Allow the cookies to cool on the baking sheet for a few minutes before transferring to a wire rack to cool completely.

Nutrition Info per Serving
- Calories: 90
- Protein: 2g
- Fat: 2g
- Carbohydrates: 18g
- Fiber: 2g
- Sugars: 8g

Serves
12 cookies

Cooking Time
20 minutes

4. Banana Bread

Ingredients
- 1 1/2 cups all-purpose flour
- 1 teaspoon baking soda
- 1/2 teaspoon ground cinnamon
- 1/4 teaspoon ground nutmeg
- 1/2 cup unsalted butter, melted
- 3/4 cup brown sugar
- 2 large eggs
- 2 cups mashed ripe bananas (about 4 bananas)
- 1 teaspoon vanilla extract

Instructions
1. Preheat the oven to 350°F (175°C). Grease a 9x5-inch loaf pan.
2. In a large bowl, whisk together the flour, baking soda, cinnamon, and nutmeg.
3. In another bowl, mix the melted butter and brown sugar until well combined.
4. Add the eggs, mashed bananas, and vanilla extract to the butter mixture and mix until smooth.
5. Pour the wet ingredients into the dry ingredients and stir until just combined. Do not overmix.
6. Pour the batter into the prepared loaf pan.
7. Bake for 55-60 minutes, or until a toothpick inserted into the center comes out clean.
8. Allow the bread to cool in the pan for 10 minutes, then transfer to a wire rack to cool completely.

Nutrition Info per Serving
- Calories: 200
- Protein: 3g
- Fat: 8g
- Carbohydrates: 30g
- Fiber: 2g
- Sugars: 15g

Serves
10 slices

Cooking Time
70 minutes

5. Boiled Carrot Sticks

Ingredients
- 4 large carrots, peeled and cut into sticks
- 4 cups water

Instructions
1. Bring the water to a boil in a large pot.
2. Add the carrot sticks and boil for 5-7 minutes, or until tender.
3. Drain the carrots and let cool slightly before serving.

Nutrition Info per Serving
- Calories: 30
- Protein: 1g
- Fat: 0g
- Carbohydrates: 7g
- Fiber: 2g
- Sugars: 4g

Serves
4

Cooking Time
10 minutes

6. Peanut Butter and Banana Sandwich

Ingredients
- 2 slices whole-grain bread
- 2 tablespoons peanut butter
- 1 ripe banana, sliced

Instructions
1. Spread the peanut butter evenly on one slice of bread.
2. Arrange the banana slices on top of the peanut butter.
3. Top with the second slice of bread.
4. Cut the sandwich in half and serve.

Nutrition Info per Serving
- Calories: 350
- Protein: 12g
- Fat: 15g
- Carbohydrates: 45g
- Fiber: 6g
- Sugars: 15g

Serves
1

Cooking Time
5 minutes

7. Smoothie Popsicles

Ingredients
- 2 cups mixed berries (strawberries, blueberries, raspberries)
- 1 banana
- 1 cup plain Greek yogurt
- 1/2 cup orange juice

Instructions
1. In a blender, combine the mixed berries, banana, Greek yogurt, and orange juice. Blend until smooth.
2. Pour the smoothie mixture into popsicle molds.
3. Insert sticks and freeze for at least 4 hours, or until solid.
4. To serve, run the popsicle molds under warm water to release the popsicles.

Nutrition Info per Serving
- Calories: 80
- Protein: 3g
- Fat: 1g
- Carbohydrates: 18g
- Fiber: 3g
- Sugars: 12g

Serves
6 popsicles

Cooking Time
10 minutes (plus freezing time)

8. Fruit Smoothie Bowl

Ingredients
- 1 cup frozen mixed berries (strawberries, blueberries, raspberries)
- 1 frozen banana
- 1/2 cup plain Greek yogurt
- 1/2 cup almond milk
- Toppings: fresh fruit, granola, chia seeds

Instructions
1. In a blender, combine the frozen berries, frozen banana, Greek yogurt, and almond milk. Blend until smooth and thick.
2. Pour the smoothie into a bowl.
3. Top with fresh fruit, granola, and chia seeds as desired.
4. Serve immediately.

Nutrition Info per Serving
- Calories: 250
- Protein: 8g
- Fat: 5g
- Carbohydrates: 45g
- Fiber: 8g
- Sugars: 25g

Serves
2

Cooking Time
10 minutes

9. Mashed Potatoes

Ingredients
- 4 large potatoes, peeled and cubed
- 1/2 cup milk (dairy or plant-based)
- 1/4 cup butter
- 1 teaspoon garlic powder

Instructions
1. Boil the potatoes in a large pot of water until tender, about 15 minutes.
2. Drain the potatoes and return them to the pot.
3. Add the milk, butter, and garlic powder. Mash until smooth.
4. Serve immediately.

Nutrition Info per Serving
- Calories: 200
- Protein: 3g
- Fat: 8g
- Carbohydrates: 30g
- Fiber: 2g
- Sugars: 2g

Serves
4

Cooking Time
20 minutes

10. Steamed Carrots

Ingredients
- 4 large carrots, peeled and sliced
- 1 cup water

Instructions
1. Bring the water to a boil in a steamer pot.
2. Add the carrot slices to the steamer basket.
3. Cover and steam for 5-7 minutes, or until tender.
4. Serve immediately.

Nutrition Info per Serving
- Calories: 30
- Protein: 1g
- Fat: 0g
- Carbohydrates: 7g
- Fiber: 2g
- Sugars: 4g

Serves
4

Cooking Time
10 minutes

11. Boiled Zucchini

Ingredients
- 4 zucchinis, sliced
- 4 cups water

Instructions
1. Bring the water to a boil in a large pot.
2. Add the zucchini slices and boil for 5-7 minutes, or until tender.
3. Drain the zucchini and let cool slightly before serving.

Nutrition Info per Serving
- Calories: 20
- Protein: 1g
- Fat: 0g
- Carbohydrates: 4g
- Fiber: 1g
- Sugars: 3g

Serves
4

Cooking Time
10 minutes

12. Steamed Spinach

Ingredients
- 1 lb fresh spinach
- 1 cup water

Instructions
1. Bring the water to a boil in a steamer pot.
2. Add the spinach to the steamer basket. 3. Cover and steam for 3-5 minutes, or until wilted.
1. Serve immediately.

Nutrition Info per Serving
- Calories: 30
- Protein: 3g
- Fat: 0g
- Carbohydrates: 5g
- Fiber: 2g
- Sugars: 0g

Serves
4

Cooking Time
10 minutes

13. Soft Polenta

Ingredients
- 1 cup polenta (coarse cornmeal)
- 4 cups water
- 1/4 cup grated Parmesan cheese
- 2 tablespoons butter
- 1 teaspoon garlic powder

Instructions
1. Bring the water to a boil in a large pot.
2. Gradually whisk in the polenta.
3. Reduce the heat to low and cook, stirring frequently, for 25-30 minutes, or until the polenta is thick and creamy.
4. Stir in the Parmesan cheese, butter, and garlic powder.
5. Serve immediately.

Nutrition Info per Serving
- Calories: 180
- Protein: 4g
- Fat: 8g
- Carbohydrates: 25g
- Fiber: 2g
- Sugars: 1g

Serves
4

Cooking Time
35 minutes

14. Creamed Corn

Ingredients
- 4 cups corn kernels (fresh or frozen)
- 1/2 cup heavy cream
- 1/4 cup milk (dairy or plant-based)
- 2 tablespoons butter
- 1 teaspoon garlic powder

Instructions
1. In a large pot, combine the corn kernels, heavy cream, milk, butter, and garlic powder.
2. Cook over medium heat, stirring frequently, until the mixture is thick and creamy, about 10-15 minutes.
3. Serve immediately.

Nutrition Info per Serving
- Calories: 200
- Protein: 4g
- Fat: 12g
- Carbohydrates: 22g
- Fiber: 3g
- Sugars: 5g

Serves
4

Cooking Time
15 minutes

15. Rice Noodles

Ingredients
- 8 oz rice noodles
- 4 cups water
- 1 tablespoon olive oil
- 1 teaspoon ground ginger

Instructions
1. Bring the water to a boil in a large pot.
2. Add the rice noodles and cook according to package instructions, usually 4-6 minutes, until tender.
3. Drain the noodles and toss with olive oil and ground ginger.
4. Serve immediately.

Nutrition Info per Serving
- Calories: 180
- Protein: 3g
- Fat: 5g
- Carbohydrates: 32g
- Fiber: 1g
- Sugars: 1g

Serves
4

Cooking Time
10 minutes

10-WEEK MEAL PLAN

Week 1
Day 1:
- **Breakfast:** Banana Oatmeal
- **Lunch:** Chicken and Rice Soup
- **Snack:** Yogurt with Honey
- **Dinner:** Baked Salmon
- **Side:** Steamed Carrots

Day 2:
- **Breakfast:** Apple Sauce Pancakes
- **Lunch:** Turkey and Vegetable Soup
- **Snack:** Peanut Butter and Banana Sandwich
- **Dinner:** Grilled Cod
- **Side:** Boiled Carrot Sticks

Day 3:
- **Breakfast:** Smoothie Bowl
- **Lunch:** Beef and Rice Soup
- **Snack:** Rice Cakes with Avocado
- **Dinner:** Baked Tilapia
- **Side:** Steamed Spinach

Day 4:
- **Breakfast:** Soft-Boiled Eggs
- **Lunch:** Chicken and Quinoa Salad
- **Snack:** Oatmeal Cookies
- **Dinner:** Beef Stew
- **Side:** Mashed Potatoes

Day 5:
- **Breakfast:** Cottage Cheese and Peaches
- **Lunch:** Pork and Rice Soup
- **Snack:** Smoothie Popsicles
- **Dinner:** Grilled Halibut
- **Side:** Boiled Zucchini

Day 6:
- **Breakfast:** Quinoa Porridge
- **Lunch:** Beef and Vegetable Bake
- **Snack:** Fruit Smoothie Bowl
- **Dinner:** Salmon Cakes
- **Side:** Soft Polenta

Day 7:
- **Breakfast:** Blueberry Muffins
- **Lunch:** Turkey Meatballs
- **Snack:** Banana Bread
- **Dinner:** Fish Tacos
- **Side:** Creamed Corn

Week 2

Day 1:
- **Breakfast:** Pumpkin Bread
- **Lunch:** Chicken and Carrot Stew
- **Snack:** Yogurt with Honey
- **Dinner:** Cod and Sweet Potato Bake
- **Side:** Steamed Carrots

Day 2:
- **Breakfast:** Avocado Toast
- **Lunch:** Pork Stew
- **Snack:** Peanut Butter and Banana Sandwich
- **Dinner:** Salmon and Spinach Frittata
- **Side:** Boiled Carrot Sticks

Day 3:
- **Breakfast:** Rice Cakes with Cottage Cheese
- **Lunch:** Ground Beef and Quinoa Bowl
- **Snack:** Oatmeal Cookies
- **Dinner:** Grilled Sole
- **Side:** Steamed Spinach

Day 4:
- **Breakfast:** Soft-Boiled Eggs
- **Lunch:** Beef and Apricot Salad
- **Snack:** Rice Cakes with Avocado
- **Dinner:** Salmon and Butternut Squash Stew
- **Side:** Mashed Potatoes

Day 5:
- **Breakfast:** Cottage Cheese and Peaches
- **Lunch:** Pork and Apricot Salad
- **Snack:** Smoothie Popsicles
- **Dinner:** Grilled Shrimp Skewers
- **Side:** Boiled Zucchini

Day 6:
- **Breakfast:** Quinoa Porridge
- **Lunch:** Beef and Pumpkin Mash
- **Snack:** Fruit Smoothie Bowl
- **Dinner:** Baked Scallops
- **Side:** Soft Polenta

Day 7:
- **Breakfast:** Blueberry Muffins
- **Lunch:** Chicken and Spinach Frittata
- **Snack:** Banana Bread
- **Dinner:** Shrimp and Rice Soup
- **Side:** Creamed Corn

Week 3

Day 1:
- **Breakfast:** Pumpkin Bread
- **Lunch:** Chicken and Quinoa Salad
- **Snack:** Yogurt with Honey
- **Dinner:** Grilled Mahi Mahi
- **Side:** Steamed Carrots

Day 2:
- **Breakfast:** Avocado Toast
- **Lunch:** Pork Meatballs
- **Snack:** Peanut Butter and Banana Sandwich
- **Dinner:** Cod and Bell Pepper Stir-Fry
- **Side:** Boiled Carrot Sticks

Day 3:
- **Breakfast:** Rice Cakes with Cottage Cheese
- **Lunch:** Beef and Mashed Potatoes
- **Snack:** Oatmeal Cookies
- **Dinner:** Grilled Halibut
- **Side:** Steamed Spinach

Day 4:
- **Breakfast:** Soft-Boiled Eggs
- **Lunch:** Turkey and Spinach Soup
- **Snack:** Rice Cakes with Avocado
- **Dinner:** Fish Tacos
- **Side:** Mashed Potatoes

Day 5:
- **Breakfast:** Cottage Cheese and Peaches
- **Lunch:** Pork and Vegetable Soup
- **Snack:** Smoothie Popsicles
- **Dinner:** Salmon and Butternut Squash Stew
- **Side:** Boiled Zucchini

Day 6:
- **Breakfast:** Quinoa Porridge
- **Lunch:** Chicken and Pumpkin Stew
- **Snack:** Fruit Smoothie Bowl
- **Dinner:** Grilled Scallops with Rice
- **Side:** Soft Polenta

Day 7:
- **Breakfast:** Blueberry Muffins
- **Lunch:** Beef and Carrot Puree
- **Snack:** Banana Bread
- **Dinner:** Shrimp and Rice Casserole
- **Side:** Creamed Corn

Week 4

Day 1:
- **Breakfast:** Pumpkin Bread
- **Lunch:** Chicken and Quinoa Salad
- **Snack:** Yogurt with Honey
- **Dinner:** Grilled Mahi Mahi
- **Side:** Steamed Carrots

Day 2:
- **Breakfast:** Avocado Toast
- **Lunch:** Pork and Soft Vegetable Casserole
- **Snack:** Peanut Butter and Banana Sandwich
- **Dinner:** Grilled Shrimp with Bell Peppers
- **Side:** Boiled Carrot Sticks

Day 3:
- **Breakfast:** Rice Cakes with Cottage Cheese
- **Lunch:** Ground Beef and Quinoa Bowl
- **Snack:** Oatmeal Cookies
- **Dinner:** Baked Flounder
- **Side:** Steamed Spinach

Day 4:
- **Breakfast:** Soft-Boiled Eggs
- **Lunch:** Beef and Apricot Salad
- **Snack:** Rice Cakes with Avocado
- **Dinner:** Salmon and Spinach Frittata
- **Side:** Mashed Potatoes

Day 5:
- **Breakfast:** Cottage Cheese and Peaches
- **Lunch:** Pork and Vegetable Bake
- **Snack:** Smoothie Popsicles
- **Dinner:** Shrimp and Zucchini Soup
- **Side:** Boiled Zucchini

Day 6:
- **Breakfast:** Quinoa Porridge
- **Lunch:** Chicken and Spinach Soup
- **Snack:** Fruit Smoothie Bowl
- **Dinner:** Grilled Scallops with Rice
- **Side:** Soft Polenta

Day 7:
- **Breakfast:** Blueberry Muffins
- **Lunch:** Beef and Mashed Potatoes
- **Snack:** Banana Bread
- **Dinner:** Baked Scallops
- **Side:** Creamed Corn

Week 5

Day 1:
- **Breakfast:** Cottage Cheese and Peaches
- **Lunch:** Beef and Vegetable Bake
- **Snack:** Yogurt with Honey
- **Dinner:** Baked Cod and Sweet Potato Bake
- **Side:** Steamed Spinach

Day 2:
- **Breakfast:** Quinoa Porridge
- **Lunch:** Pork Stew
- **Snack:** Smoothie Popsicles
- **Dinner:** Grilled Mahi Mahi
- **Side:** Mashed Potatoes

Day 3:
- **Breakfast:** Blueberry Muffins
- **Lunch:** Chicken and Pumpkin Stew
- **Snack:** Rice Cakes with Avocado
- **Dinner:** Baked Tilapia
- **Side:** Boiled Carrot Sticks

Day 4:
- **Breakfast:** Pumpkin Bread
- **Lunch:** Beef and Carrot Puree
- **Snack:** Peanut Butter and Banana Sandwich
- **Dinner:** Grilled Shrimp Skewers
- **Side:** Soft Polenta

Day 5:
- **Breakfast:** Avocado Toast
- **Lunch:** Turkey and Apricot Salad
- **Snack:** Fruit Smoothie Bowl
- **Dinner:** Salmon Cakes
- **Side:** Creamed Corn

Day 6:
- **Breakfast:** Rice Cakes with Cottage Cheese
- **Lunch:** Pork and Rice Soup
- **Snack:** Banana Bread
- **Dinner:** Grilled Halibut
- **Side:** Steamed Carrots

Day 7:
- **Breakfast:** Soft-Boiled Eggs
- **Lunch:** Chicken and Spinach Soup
- **Snack:** Oatmeal Cookies
- **Dinner:** Shrimp and Zucchini Soup
- **Side:** Boiled Zucchini

Week 6

Day 1:
- **Breakfast:** Banana Oatmeal
- **Lunch:** Pork and Vegetable Bake
- **Snack:** Smoothie Popsicles
- **Dinner:** Grilled Cod
- **Side:** Steamed Spinach

Day 2:
- **Breakfast:** Apple Sauce Pancakes
- **Lunch:** Beef Stew
- **Snack:** Rice Cakes with Avocado
- **Dinner:** Baked Flounder
- **Side:** Mashed Potatoes

Day 3:
- **Breakfast:** Smoothie Bowl
- **Lunch:** Chicken and Quinoa Salad
- **Snack:** Peanut Butter and Banana Sandwich
- **Dinner:** Grilled Sole
- **Side:** Boiled Carrot Sticks

Day 4:
- **Breakfast:** Cottage Cheese and Peaches
- **Lunch:** Beef and Rice Soup
- **Snack:** Yogurt with Honey
- **Dinner:** Grilled Shrimp with Bell Peppers
- **Side:** Soft Polenta

Day 5:
- **Breakfast:** Quinoa Porridge
- **Lunch:** Turkey and Vegetable Soup
- **Snack:** Fruit Smoothie Bowl
- **Dinner:** Baked Scallops
- **Side:** Creamed Corn

Day 6:
- **Breakfast:** Blueberry Muffins
- **Lunch:** Pork and Apricot Salad
- **Snack:** Rice Cakes with Cottage Cheese
- **Dinner:** Grilled Halibut
- **Side:** Steamed Carrots

Day 7:
- **Breakfast:** Pumpkin Bread
- **Lunch:** Beef and Pumpkin Mash
- **Snack:** Oatmeal Cookies
- **Dinner:** Salmon and Butternut Squash Stew
- **Side:** Boiled Zucchini

Week 7

Day 1:
- **Breakfast:** Avocado Toast
- **Lunch:** Chicken and Carrot Stew
- **Snack:** Smoothie Popsicles
- **Dinner:** Grilled Mahi Mahi
- **Side:** Mashed Potatoes

Day 2:
- **Breakfast:** Rice Cakes with Cottage Cheese
- **Lunch:** Pork Stew
- **Snack:** Peanut Butter and Banana Sandwich
- **Dinner:** Grilled Shrimp Skewers
- **Side:** Boiled Carrot Sticks

Day 3:
- **Breakfast:** Soft-Boiled Eggs
- **Lunch:** Beef and Mashed Potatoes
- **Snack:** Fruit Smoothie Bowl
- **Dinner:** Baked Tilapia
- **Side:** Steamed Spinach

Day 4:
- **Breakfast:** Cottage Cheese and Peaches
- **Lunch:** Pork and Vegetable Soup
- **Snack:** Rice Cakes with Avocado
- **Dinner:** Salmon Cakes
- **Side:** Soft Polenta

Day 5:
- **Breakfast:** Quinoa Porridge
- **Lunch:** Beef and Vegetable Bake
- **Snack:** Banana Bread
- **Dinner:** Baked Flounder
- **Side:** Creamed Corn

Day 6:
- **Breakfast:** Blueberry Muffins
- **Lunch:** Chicken and Spinach Soup
- **Snack:** Yogurt with Honey
- **Dinner:** Grilled Cod
- **Side:** Boiled Zucchini

Day 7:
- **Breakfast:** Pumpkin Bread
- **Lunch:** Ground Beef and Quinoa Bowl
- **Snack:** Oatmeal Cookies
- **Dinner:** Grilled Sole
- **Side:** Steamed Carrots

Week 8

Day 1:
- **Breakfast:** Avocado Toast
- **Lunch:** Chicken and Quinoa Salad
- **Snack:** Smoothie Popsicles
- **Dinner:** Baked Scallops
- **Side:** Mashed Potatoes

Day 2:
- **Breakfast:** Rice Cakes with Cottage Cheese
- **Lunch:** Pork and Rice Soup
- **Snack:** Peanut Butter and Banana Sandwich
- **Dinner:** Grilled Halibut
- **Side:** Boiled Carrot Sticks

Day 3:
- **Breakfast:** Soft-Boiled Eggs
- **Lunch:** Beef and Apricot Salad
- **Snack:** Fruit Smoothie Bowl
- **Dinner:** Grilled Mahi Mahi
- **Side:** Steamed Spinach

Day 4:
- **Breakfast:** Cottage Cheese and Peaches
- **Lunch:** Beef and Carrot Puree
- **Snack:** Rice Cakes with Avocado
- **Dinner:** Grilled Shrimp with Bell Peppers
- **Side:** Soft Polenta

Day 5:
- **Breakfast:** Quinoa Porridge
- **Lunch:** Chicken and Pumpkin Stew
- **Snack:** Banana Bread
- **Dinner:** Baked Tilapia
- **Side:** Creamed Corn

Day 6:
- **Breakfast:** Blueberry Muffins
- **Lunch:** Pork and Vegetable Bake
- **Snack:** Yogurt with Honey
- **Dinner:** Salmon and Butternut Squash Stew
- **Side:** Boiled Zucchini

Day 7:
- **Breakfast:** Pumpkin Bread
- **Lunch:** Turkey and Spinach Soup
- **Snack:** Oatmeal Cookies
- **Dinner:** Grilled Shrimp Skewers
- **Side:** Steamed Carrots

Week 9

Day 1:
- **Breakfast:** Peach Yogurt Parfait
- **Lunch:** Beef and Vegetable Bake
- **Snack:** Rice Cakes with Cottage Cheese
- **Dinner:** Grilled Halibut
- **Side:** Boiled Zucchini

Day 2:
- **Breakfast:** Egg Muffins
- **Lunch:** Pork and Rice Soup
- **Snack:** Smoothie Popsicles
- **Dinner:** Grilled Mahi Mahi
- **Side:** Steamed Carrots

Day 3:
- **Breakfast:** Soft Cheese Omelette
- **Lunch:** Ground Beef and Quinoa Bowl
- **Snack:** Peanut Butter and Banana Sandwich
- **Dinner:** Baked Salmon
- **Side:** Mashed Potatoes

Day 4:
- **Breakfast:** Peach Smoothie
- **Lunch:** Beef Stew
- **Snack:** Fruit Smoothie Bowl
- **Dinner:** Grilled Shrimp with Bell Peppers
- **Side:** Soft Polenta

Day 5:
- **Breakfast:** Cinnamon Toast
- **Lunch:** Chicken and Spinach Soup
- **Snack:** Banana Bread
- **Dinner:** Baked Tilapia
- **Side:** Creamed Corn

Day 6:
- **Breakfast:** Baked Oatmeal
- **Lunch:** Pork and Apricot Salad
- **Snack:** Yogurt with Honey
- **Dinner:** Grilled Sole
- **Side:** Steamed Spinach

Day 7:
- **Breakfast:** Soft Cheese and Crackers
- **Lunch:** Chicken and Pumpkin Stew
- **Snack:** Oatmeal Cookies
- **Dinner:** Grilled Cod
- **Side:** Boiled Carrot Sticks

Week 10

Day 1:
- **Breakfast:** Egg and Cheese Quesadilla
- **Lunch:** Beef and Rice Soup
- **Snack:** Rice Cakes with Avocado
- **Dinner:** Baked Flounder
- **Side:** Steamed Carrots

Day 2:
- **Breakfast:** Creamy Semolina
- **Lunch:** Chicken and Quinoa Salad
- **Snack:** Smoothie Popsicles
- **Dinner:** Grilled Halibut
- **Side:** Boiled Zucchini

Day 3:
- **Breakfast:** Banana Oatmeal
- **Lunch:** Pork Stew
- **Snack:** Peanut Butter and Banana Sandwich
- **Dinner:** Grilled Shrimp Skewers
- **Side:** Mashed Potatoes

Day 4:
- **Breakfast:** Apple Sauce Pancakes
- **Lunch:** Beef and Carrot Puree
- **Snack:** Fruit Smoothie Bowl
- **Dinner:** Baked Salmon
- **Side:** Creamed Corn

Day 5:
- **Breakfast:** Smoothie Bowl
- **Lunch:** Turkey and Vegetable Soup
- **Snack:** Banana Bread
- **Dinner:** Grilled Mahi Mahi
- **Side:** Steamed Spinach

Day 6:
- **Breakfast:** Soft-Boiled Eggs
- **Lunch:** Ground Beef and Quinoa Bowl
- **Snack:** Yogurt with Honey
- **Dinner:** Baked Tilapia
- **Side:** Boiled Carrot Sticks

Day 7:
- **Breakfast:** Peach Yogurt Parfait
- **Lunch:** Chicken and Spinach Soup
- **Snack:** Oatmeal Cookies
- **Dinner:** Grilled Shrimp with Bell Peppers
- **Side:** Soft Polenta

MEAL PLANNER JOURNAL

	BREAKFAST	LUNCH	DINNER	SNACKS
MON				
TUE				
WED				
THU				
FRI				
SAT				
SUN				

What were your eating habits like before your colostomy surgery? How do you anticipate they will change as you start the colostomy diet?

MEAL PLANNER JOURNAL

	BREAKFAST	LUNCH	DINNER	SNACKS
MON				
TUE				
WED				
THU				
FRI				
SAT				
SUN				

What foods have you been advised to avoid following your colostomy surgery, and why?

MEAL PLANNER JOURNAL

	BREAKFAST	LUNCH	DINNER	SNACKS
MON				
TUE				
WED				
THU				
FRI				
SAT				
SUN				

What are your top three dietary goals while following the colostomy diet? How do you plan to achieve them?

MEAL PLANNER JOURNAL

	BREAKFAST	LUNCH	DINNER	SNACKS
MON				
TUE				
WED				
THU				
FRI				
SAT				
SUN				

Describe a typical day's meals and snacks that align with the colostomy diet. How do you ensure you get a balanced diet?

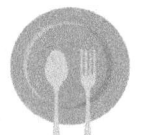

MEAL PLANNER JOURNAL

	BREAKFAST	LUNCH	DINNER	SNACKS
MON				
TUE				
WED				
THU				
FRI				
SAT				
SUN				

How much water do you aim to drink daily, and why is staying hydrated important for colostomy patients?

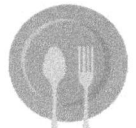

MEAL PLANNER JOURNAL

	BREAKFAST	LUNCH	DINNER	SNACKS
MON				
TUE				
WED				
THU				
FRI				
SAT				
SUN				

What foods have you noticed cause discomfort or digestive issues since your surgery? How do you plan to manage these triggers?

MEAL PLANNER JOURNAL

	BREAKFAST	LUNCH	DINNER	SNACKS
MON				
TUE				
WED				
THU				
FRI				
SAT				
SUN				

How comfortable are you with cooking at home? What are some easy and colostomy-friendly recipes you plan to try?

MEAL PLANNER JOURNAL

	BREAKFAST	LUNCH	DINNER	SNACKS
MON				
TUE				
WED				
THU				
FRI				
SAT				
SUN				

What strategies will you use to make colostomy-friendly choices when dining out or ordering takeout?

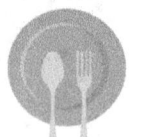

MEAL PLANNER JOURNAL

	BREAKFAST	LUNCH	DINNER	SNACKS
MON				
TUE				
WED				
THU				
FRI				
SAT				
SUN				

How can keeping a food journal help you track your diet and identify any problematic foods? What specific details will you include in your journal?

MEAL PLANNER JOURNAL

	BREAKFAST	LUNCH	DINNER	SNACKS
MON				
TUE				
WED				
THU				
FRI				
SAT				
SUN				

How will you handle cravings for foods that might not be suitable for your colostomy diet?

MEAL PLANNER JOURNAL

	BREAKFAST	LUNCH	DINNER	SNACKS
MON				
TUE				
WED				
THU				
FRI				
SAT				
SUN				

What foods or beverages have you been advised to avoid to reduce gas and odor? What strategies will you use to manage these issues?

MEAL PLANNER JOURNAL

	BREAKFAST	LUNCH	DINNER	SNACKS
MON				
TUE				
WED				
THU				
FRI				
SAT				
SUN				

What specific information will you look for on nutrition labels to ensure the foods you choose are suitable for your colostomy diet?

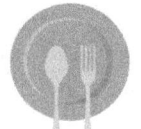

MEAL PLANNER JOURNAL

	BREAKFAST	LUNCH	DINNER	SNACKS
MON				
TUE				
WED				
THU				
FRI				
SAT				
SUN				

Who can you rely on for support and advice as you adjust to your new diet? How will you involve them in your journey?

Scan the QR code to Get Your Downloadable E-book with Full Color Pictures

www.ingramcontent.com/pod-product-compliance
Lightning Source LLC
Chambersburg PA
CBHW082206220526
45470CB00010B/3057